RODALE'S
ESSENTIAL
HERBAL
HANDBOOKS

Herbal Remedies

DOZENS OF SAFE, EFFECTIVE TREATMENTS TO GROW AND MAKE

Kathleen Fisher

Rodale Press, Inc.
Emmaus, Pennsylvania

for JoAnne

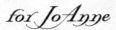

OUR PURPOSE

We inspire and enable people to improve their lives and the world around them.

Storey Books:
Editor: Gwen W. Steege
Text Designer: Eugenie Seidenberg Delaney
Cover Designer: Meredith Maker
Text Illustrators: Illustrations by Beverly Duncan, except those by Charles Joslin, pages 3, 29, 32, 34, 35, 41, 57 (top), 63, 116; Sarah Brill, pages 33, 44, 54, 55, 57 (bottom), 59, 64 (bottom left, middle), 66, 68, 110, 130; Alison Kolesar, pages 38, 113; Brigita Fuhrmann, pages 61, 65, 74; Judy Eliason, page 64 (bottom right); and Mallory Lake, pages 67, 69
Production Assistants: Susan Bernier and Erin Lincourt
Indexer: Susan Olason

Rodale Press Garden Books:
Executive Editor: Ellen Phillips
Editor: Karen Costello Soltys
Executive Creative Director: Christin Gangi
Art Director and Cover Designer: Patricia Field
Cover Illustrator: Mia Bosna
Studio Manager: Leslie Keefe
Manufacturing Manager: Mark Krahforst

For questions or comments concerning the editorial content of this book, please write to:

Rodale Press, Inc.
Book Readers' Service
33 East Minor Street
Emmaus, PA 18098

For more information about Rodale Press and the books and magazines we publish, visit our World Wide Web site at:
http://www.rodalepress.com

Library of Congress Cataloging-in-Publication Data

Fisher, Kathleen
  Herbal remedies / Kathleen Fisher.
    p.   cm. — (Rodale's essential herbal handbooks)
  Includes bibliographical references (p.   ) and index.
  ISBN 0–87596–816–3 (hardcover : alk. paper)
  ISBN 0–87596–831–7 (pbk. : alk. paper)
  1. Herbs—Therapeutic use.   2. Materia medica, Vegetable.
  3. Medicinal plants.   I. Title.   II. Series.
  RM666.H33 F574 1999
  615'.321—dc21   99–6019

Distributed in the book trade by St. Martin's Press
Printed in the United States
2 4 6 8 10 9 7 5 3 1   hardcover
2 4 6 8 10 9 7 5 3 1   paperback

Contents

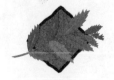

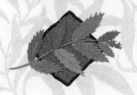

CHAPTER 1

HERBS ~
to Your Health

Welcome to the wonderful world of healing herbs! If you're a gardener, you may grow some thyme for your cooking, or lavender for its refreshing scent. But did you know that thyme can also cure indigestion, stop coughs, relieve pain, and kill germs? And that lovely lavender can reduce stress or take the heat out of a sunburn? Other, more flamboyant garden perennials, as well as some trees and shrubs, are also healing herbs. Both the tall, feathery-flowered meadowsweet and the dramatic white willow tree contain the same powerful painkiller that is in aspirin. And witch hazel, a small native tree that brings welcome color to late winter gardens, treats all kinds of discomforts, from sore muscles to tired eyes. Once you start exploring herbs, you may want to create an entire landscape of healing plants!

Herbs have a long tradition as healers, one that many of us — scientists and laypeople alike — are today looking at with fresh curiosity and a growing respect. As you will see, it's easy to become a part of this tradition, learning which herbs to use and how to use them to prevent and treat the discomforts, injuries, and illnesses that afflict us all. And as you learn, you will become more confident that herbs are not only effective but also safe for you and your family.

This book is designed to guide your own exploration of this fascinating subject. There are three basics that you'll be working with: the methods of making herbal medicines, the herbs themselves, and the various symptoms you may need to treat.

Chapter 2, "Herbal Healing Formulas," describes the various techniques you'll use to prepare your herbal medicines. In Chapter 3, "Essential Healing Herbs A to Z," you'll find 32 terrific herbs that you'll want to have on hand for the most common health problems. I've chosen them because they are both easy to find — either on the shelf at a health food store or pharmacy, or growing in your garden — and particularly effective. Most of these herbs have stood up to hundreds of years of folk use and more important, to the rigors of modern science. In Chapter 4, "Growing Healing Herbs," you'll learn how easy it is to grow, harvest, and store a year's supply of healing herbs. Chapter 5, "Symptoms and Remedies," is a directory of common ailments and symptoms with the best herbal treatments. You can look up more than 40 common symptoms and learn what experts consider the best herbs for treating them.

USING HERBS AS MEDICINE

Several herbs have made headlines in the past year or so, including three in particular — St.-John's-wort for depression, echinacea for colds and flu, and ginkgo for memory. Herbal medicine is definitely moving out of health food stores and into the mainstream.

Our increased awareness of our environment also links us more closely to its benefits. When we hear that lifesaving rainforest plants, such as Madagascar periwinkle *(Catharanthus roseus),* can cure

What Is an Herb?

Botanists say that an herb is a plant without any woody parts that disappears in the winter. But for herbalists, crafters, and others, an herb is simply any plant that is useful. Trees like ginkgo (used for cardiovascular health) and witch hazel (a popular astringent wash) are herbs. Roses make the list because of their hips, so rich in vitamin C, and so does the homely "weed" plantain, useful for skin injuries, sore throats, and hemorrhoids. Fruits and vegetables can be herbs. If you have high blood pressure, for instance, carrots, peas, and pineapple can help prevent stroke. Spicy red peppers can alleviate allergy symptoms and ease pain. What a great way to take your medicine!

leukemia and Hodgkin's disease, we recognize our dependence on the power of plants. And we're inspired to support efforts to control the rate at which plant species disappear from earth.

Our relationship with plants is as old as time, and we've renewed that relationship by turning to our gardens in record numbers. For many of us, the garden is both a blank canvas where we can be creative and a chapel in which to find solace and spiritual restoration. But did you know that merely looking at plants has a positive effect on your health? It lowers blood pressure, much as meditation might. Growing herbs for health brings yet another dimension to what has become the nation's most popular pastime.

We can use herbs to relax, drinking chamomile tea before bed or putting a few drops of lavender oil in the bath. We can take herbs to treat discomfort, chewing some feverfew leaves for a migraine headache. But the real beauty of herbs is in using them for prevention. When our ancestors took a spring tonic of tender dandelion leaves and some powdered sassafras or sarsaparilla root, they knew what they were doing!

German
Chamomile

Because you'll be making your own choices, exploring herbal remedies is a liberating experience. You may wish to grow many medicinal herbs in your own garden or purchase dried leaves or berries at a health food store, or you may decide you like the convenience of bottled pills and tinctures. Try just one new herb at a time, to make sure that you don't have any allergies or other side effects, and switch to an alternative if you have any unpleasant symptoms. Although there are a few herbs that are considered unwise to take for long periods, you will take most for only a day or two. Be alert to any changes in your health if you decide to introduce an herb into your daily regimen for long-term benefits. Most herbal medicines are extremely gentle. In fact, they are probably most effective not as "quick cures," but when we make them part of our regular routine, along with eating more fruits and whole grains, and drinking more water. Like good nutrition, fresh air, and exercise, herbs deserve to be a part of every healthy lifestyle. Herbs to your health!

Safety First

Most of the herbs listed in this book are very safe. Still, you need to think of them as drugs and use them with common sense.

- Are you pregnant? You should definitely avoid a few herbs, including barberry, feverfew, tansy, chervil, and mountain mint.
- Do you have allergies? Some herbs, such as chamomile and calendula, are closely related to ragweed and can cause hay-fever-type reactions.
- Are you taking prescription drugs regularly? Some herbs interact with drugs and food, or with other herbs. Discuss your interest in herbs with your doctor.
- Are you having any unpleasant reaction to taking an herb? If you feel dizzy or your stomach is upset, the herb may be causing side effects, and you should stop taking it.
- Are you following the recommended dose? Remember, taking twice as much of something isn't twice as good for you!

CHAPTER 2

HERBAL
Healing
Formulas

As with any subject that's new, information about herbal medicine may refer to terms and techniques that you're not familiar with. You're about to discover, however, that procedures like making an infusion or a decoction are just as simple as boiling an egg. In fact, once you get comfortable with herbs you won't always need recipes. The vast majority are so safe that you can use a pinch of this and a pinch of that, just as you would when spicing up your spaghetti sauce. Sometimes you can even add a few leaves or flowers to food to benefit from medicinal herbs.

If you're taking herbs medicinally for the first time, or if you want to be sure you're taking all you can for an ache or pain without overdoing it, you'll feel a lot more comfortable when you've mastered the basic terms and techniques.

DECIDING WHETHER TO MAKE
OR BUY YOUR HERBAL MEDICINE

The world of healing herbs offers plenty of options, both in the forms your medicine can take and whether you should make the product or purchase it.

Some herbs are simple to grow and use, but there are others that you will need or want to buy. Some herbs won't grow in your climate, and some, like ginkgo, must be processed with professional equipment. Unless you have a big garden, you may not be able to harvest enough fresh herbs to get you through the winter, or maybe you won't want to sacrifice the echinacea in your butterfly garden to collect the roots needed for medicine. In other cases, as with calendula, it will be a toss-up, because the herb is a snap to grow and prepare, but is also easy to buy in many different forms. If you like making your own medicines but don't want to grow your own herbs, you can find bulk herbs in many health food stores and organic groceries.

Although only you can decide what is best and most convenient for your own and your family's needs, it's likely you'll keep a combination of purchased and homemade remedies on hand, along with

Don't Forget to Label!

If you've ever sown seeds indoors in late winter and forgotten to label your flats, you remember how frustrated you felt. Well, labels are much more important when making herbal medicines. Have a label ready as soon as you bottle an infusion or tincture. Include the plant name and date, and a note on suggested doses.

Have fun with your labels! Snip a photograph of the plant from a mail-order catalog, or use felt-tip markers to give the label your own logo. If you're computer savvy, try your hand at creating your own logo and label using one of the many programs designed for the purpose.

some fundamental ingredients and supplies for making last-minute formulations. This chapter describes the types of formulas you can make — from tinctures that can be stored for up to two years, to more simple infusions (teas) and ointments. You'll also learn the basic techniques you'll need for making all these types of remedies. And, at the end of the chapter, you'll find some recommendations for what to include in your own herbal medicine chest.

EQUIPMENT AND SUPPLIES FOR MAKING HERBAL REMEDIES

Having the right equipment on hand is easier than you may think. Chances are that you already have most everything you'll need in your kitchen cabinets. If not, it's fairly basic stuff, easy and inexpensive to acquire from most grocery stores or houseware departments.

Nonaluminum cookware. Use saucepans made of stainless steel, enamel, or glassware. Evidence suggests that aluminum may release toxins that herbs can absorb. A double boiler is especially useful. If you don't have one, though, you can improvise by fitting a saucepan with a bowl or smaller pan that nestles into it, with the bowl's bottom an inch or so above water in the saucepan.

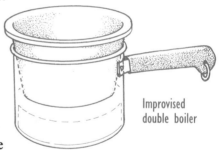

Improvised double boiler

Airtight storage containers. They should be dark glass or ceramic. Clear glass will expose your herbs to light, which decreases their potency. Plastic containers may let air through and absorb chemicals from the herbs, so you'll want to avoid them.

Kitchen scales. Sometimes called dieter's scales, these weigh items up to a pound and are useful when recipes list herb amounts in grams or ounces.

Measuring cups and spoons. Most of the recipes in this book are given in these measures.

Coffee grinder or mortar and pestle. You can use either of these to grind up seeds, stems, and dried roots.

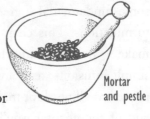
Mortar and pestle

Plastic strainer or sieve. You will usually need to strain herbs out after you cook or steep them.

OTHER HELPFUL ITEMS

Funnel. A funnel will make it easier to pour herbal mixtures into storage bottles.

Jelly bags. They're useful for squeezing fluid from herbs. Look for jelly bags in the canning section of your supermarket or hardware store. You can also use a piece of clean, porous fabric, such as light-weight cotton or three or four layers of cheesecloth.

Tea kettle and glass or ceramic teapot. You'll find this pair convenient for heating water and steeping herbs.

The Search for Containers

Once you start collecting containers for your herbs, it may become an obsession! It's important to use dark-colored glass, so your herbs won't be exposed to light. Craft stores and even groceries sell large, colored bottles with stoppers, used often for herbal vinegars. Some of them have taps near the bottom, which you'll find handy for tonic wines.

I haunt flea markets and garage sales looking for old medicine bottles. I've even found useful bottles while beachcombing. Just be sure to sterilize your finds, and check that they have no cracks or chips. If you can locate bottles with droppers, they will help you measure out your tinctures.

MAKING MIXTURES TO TREAT INTERNAL PROBLEMS

There are several different ways to prepare herbs to take internally, including infusions, decoctions, tinctures, syrups, tonic wines, and capsules. You make infusions and decoctions by steeping or boiling herbs in water. These may be made with fresh or dried herbs, but the preparations themselves don't keep for more than a day or two in the refrigerator. To prepare tinctures, you combine herbs with alcohol. Although tinctures take longer to make, they also keep much longer, so you can make them ahead of time to have ready when discomfort strikes unexpectedly. Syrups, too, take a bit more work to prepare, but are especially useful for sore throats or to disguise bitter herbs. Tonic wines, like tinctures, are easy to prepare, but require time to extract the benefits of the herbs. They aren't as strong as other preparations, but you may find them an enjoyable way to take your healthful herbs.

Dry versus Fresh

The proportions in the following recipes are for dried herbs. If you're using fresh herbs, use twice as much as what's called for. The exception to the rule is when you're making a tincture. Then you'll need to use only 50 percent more.

Infusions

Some herbalists use the word *tea* when talking about either an infusion or a decoction. Using these more specific words helps remind you, first, that you are drinking herbs as medicine, not as thirst-quenchers, and, second, how each one is made. You make an infusion with the softer parts of an herb that grow above ground — stems, leaves, and/or flowers. Because they are soft, you don't need to cook them over heat. Proportions of herb to water vary slightly depending on the herb you are using, but usually 1 to 3 teaspoons per cup of water is recommended. Because of the short storage time of infusions, you will usually make only one to six cups at a time.

BASIC RECIPE FOR AN INFUSION

1. Place the herbs in a teapot.
2. In a kettle or saucepan, bring the water to the boiling point, turn off the heat, and pour the water over the herbs.

What You Need

1–3 teaspoons dried herbs
1 cup water

3. Cover the teapot, and let the herbs steep for 10 to 20 minutes.
4. Strain the liquid into a cup for immediate use, or into a storage container.

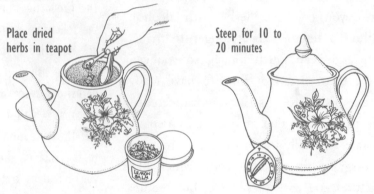

Place dried herbs in teapot

Steep for 10 to 20 minutes

Storage. Two days in the refrigerator.

Dose. For most herbs, unless otherwise directed, you can drink one to three cups a day to relieve discomfort.

Decoctions

Because decoctions use the tough parts of an herb (bark, roots, or dry berries), you treat them in a slightly different manner from the way you would treat delicate flowers. A decoction is similar to an infusion except that you simmer or boil the herbs instead of simply steeping them. The proportions of the herb to water vary slightly depending on the herb you are using. In this book, recipes usually describe decoctions in terms of number of teaspoons of dried herb per cup of water. Like infusions, decoctions have a short storage time, so you will usually make only one to six cups at a time.

BASIC RECIPE FOR A DECOCTION

1. Place herbs and water in a saucepan. Bring to a boil; then lower the heat and let the mixture simmer for 15 to 30 minutes. (Some recipes suggest a shorter simmering time.) Cover the cooking pan to keep the water from evaporating, along with some of the potency of the herb. Keep an eye on your pot during this period to make sure the water hasn't simmered away. Turn off the heat.

2. **If you wish to use the mixture immediately,** strain the liquid into a tea cup or mug.

3. **If you wish to store the mixture,** allow it to cool. Be sure to leave the lid on the pan while the mixture is cooling. Strain liquid into a storage container.

What You Need

1 tablespoon dried herbs

2 cups water

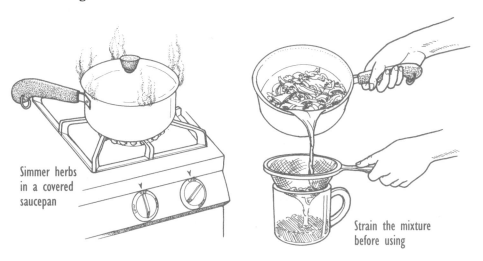

Simmer herbs in a covered saucepan

Strain the mixture before using

Storage. Two days in the refrigerator.

Dose. Unless otherwise indicated in the information about the specific herb you're using, you can usually drink one to three cups a day to relieve discomfort.

Tinctures

Tinctures are made with alcohol. Most people use vodka, but you can also use grain alcohol (198 proof, compared to vodka's 40 to 100 proof). Some people use rum or brandy when they make tinctures with bitter herbs, to help disguise the taste. If you're preparing a tincture for use by children, recovered alcoholics, or others who should avoid alcohol, you can substitute cider vinegar for the alcohol. Unfortunately, vinegar doesn't extract some herbs as efficiently as alcohol does. Tinctures are more concentrated and keep longer than infusions and decoctions.

Safety first. Never use denatured or rubbing alcohol for this purpose. It is highly toxic and should never be taken internally.

BASIC RECIPE FOR A TINCTURE

What You Need

1 ounce dried herbs
5 ounces alcohol

1. Combine the ingredients in a glass or ceramic jar with a nonmetallic lid.
2. Set the jar in a cool, dark place for two to six weeks. Shake the jar periodically to help the alcohol extract the herb's active ingredients.
3. Strain the liquid into another clean jar, and store.

Storage. Two years.

Dose. You will usually take ½ to 1 teaspoon of a tincture, no more than three times a day.

Take a Deep Breath

You can bask in the benefits of herbs while you're cooking them by inhaling their fragrant steam. If you want a powerful hit of steam to soothe sinuses, for instance, run your bathroom sink full of hot water, add a few drops of eucalyptus oil or a handful of mint leaves, and make a "tent" over your head with a towel. A steam tent might also help teenage acne. It opens pores and makes skin more amenable to cleansing. Substitute a handful of calendula flowers for the eucalyptus.

Syrups

The bitterness of some herbs serves natural purposes: to keep us from overdosing, as well as to stimulate digestive juices. Unfortunately, the bitterness is no help to us if we turn up our noses at a medicine's taste and refuse to take it. Syrups are a good alternative way to prepare some mixtures, and one that can extend the storage life of the herb. And for colds or flus, syrups can also soothe a sore throat.

Safety first. Honey should never be given to children younger than a year. Honey sometimes contains botulism spores, and although the count is so low that it doesn't affect older children and adults, the digestive systems of very young children aren't mature enough to handle the spores.

BASIC RECIPE FOR A SYRUP

1. Combine the infusion or decoction and the honey or sugar in a saucepan.
2. Heat gently until the sugar or honey has completely dissolved.
3. Pour into a clean glass or ceramic container.

What You Need
1 part herbal infusion or decoction
1 part honey or unrefined sugar

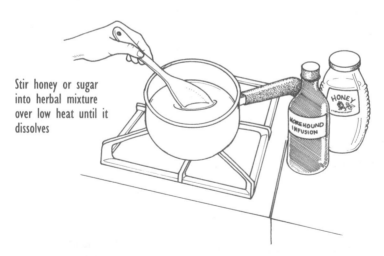

Stir honey or sugar into herbal mixture over low heat until it dissolves

Storage. Three to six months in the refrigerator.

Dose. You may use 1 to 2 teaspoons of syrup up to three times a day.

Tonic Wines

A really relaxing way to consume herbs is in tonic wines, and they're easy to make. Because the wine ferments the herb, however, it loses some of its medicinal value. If you have a vinegar vat, the tap makes it easy to draw off the liquid.

BASIC RECIPE FOR A TONIC WINE

1. Measure the herbs into a vat or ceramic jar, and add the wine. Be sure that the herbs are completely covered by liquid. Steep the mixture for at least two weeks.

2. Strain or draw off as needed.

Storage. Up to four months, away from a heat source. Check the wine frequently for mold, and if any forms, throw the mixture away.

Dose. Drink a small glass before dinner. Herbal wines are an especially good way to dispense dried roots like ginseng *(Panax quinquefolius, P. ginseng, Eleutherococus senticosus)* and Chinese angelica *(Angelica sinensis).*

> ## What You Need
> 3 ounces dried herb leaves or 2 teaspoons powdered root
> 1 liter red wine

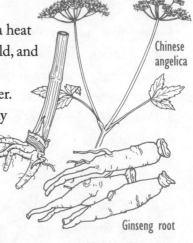

Chinese angelica

Ginseng root

Capsules

If you'd rather not drink your medicines, you can buy or make capsules. One advantage of capsules is that they are easier than liquids to take along to work or when traveling.

BASIC TECHNIQUE FOR FILLING CAPSULES

1. Powder the dry herbs by grinding them in a coffee grinder or with a mortar and pestle.

> ## What You Need
> Gelatin capsules, size 00
> ½ gram herb for each capsule

2. Scoop the powder into the capsules by bringing the halves of the capsules together.

3. Store capsules in a clean jar, tightly covered.

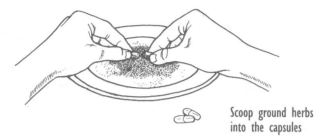

Scoop ground herbs into the capsules

Storage. Three to four months.

Dose. Swallow a capsule with water. Or, open it and sprinkle on food, or use it to make an infusion or tincture.

MAKING MIXTURES TO TREAT EXTERNAL PROBLEMS

You don't have to swallow herbs to enjoy their healing powers. Poultices and compresses will heal and soothe skin injuries with little or no preparation. Herbal oils, ointments, and salves are more work, but will let you exercise creativity and give the restorative benefit of human touch when you apply them with your fingers.

Poultices

If you're hiking in the woods and lose a fight with a briar patch, you can help stop the bleeding by pressing a handful of crushed wild geranium *(Geranium maculatum)* leaves against the cut. That bunch of leaves is actually a poultice. At home and with more time, you can make a more sophisticated version. You can use fresh, dry, or powdered herbs to make a poultice. The goal is to chop them finely and get them damp enough that they release their volatile oils. Fresh herbs will supply some of their own moisture.

The amount you make will depend on the size of the injured area. Depending on the type of injury, you might want to make enough so that you can change the poultice several times, with two or three hours between changes. If possible, you can wrap the area with a piece of gauze to hold the poultice in place.

BASIC METHOD FOR MAKING A POULTICE

Method 1. Put the herbs in a food processor or blender, and give them a spin, adding a bit of water to create a sticky paste.

Method 2. For a warm poultice or if you are using dried or powdered herbs, put the herbs in a saucepan. Barely cover them with water, and simmer carefully for 2 or 3 minutes. Allow to cool slightly before applying.

Method 3. For plants with large, tough leaves (such as mature comfrey), boil water in a saucepan and then, holding the leaves with tongs, dip the leaves into the water to soften them.

Storage. Use poultices fresh; they do not store.

Use. Apply a poultice to insect bites and stings, bruises, swelling, cuts, and scrapes. Wrap the area with a piece of gauze to hold the poultice in place. Generally, warm poultices are soothing for muscle sprains, while cold ones are helpful for bruises.

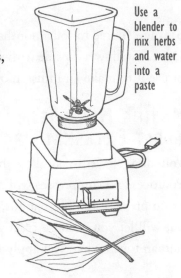

Use a blender to mix herbs and water into a paste

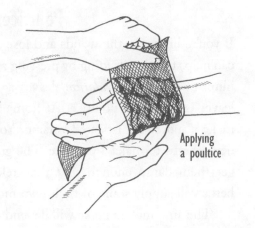

Applying a poultice

Compresses

The approach is similar to a poultice, but you use a liquid solution instead of whole herbs. Traditionally, a compress is hot, but sometimes, especially for a headache, a cold compress may feel better.

BASIC METHOD FOR MAKING A COMPRESS

1. Soak a clean cotton cloth (such as a wash cloth or a piece of an old tee shirt) in the infusion, decoction, or diluted tincture.
2. Wring out the cloth so that it is not dripping, and fold it 2 or 3 times.

Use. Apply damp compress to injured or problem area. Compresses are wonderful for sore joints and muscles, rashes and other skin irritations, burning or tired eyes, and cuts and scrapes. Replenish hot compresses when they cool (or cold compresses when they warm up), if desired.

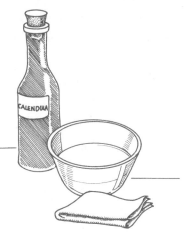

Herbal Oils

To make homemade oils, most people use a hot process because it's faster, but the cold process may be gentler for infusing flowers. The cold method of preparation is a lot like making sun tea — only slower. Using a large, clear glass container is important, because you want the heat and light of the sun to "cook" your mix. Use a high-quality cooking oil, such as extra virgin olive, safflower, or grapeseed oil. Herbal oil infusions are useful for massages to relieve pain or tension, and also as a treatment for skin problems. None are for internal use.

Safety first. Don't confuse herbal oil infusions with essential oils, which are pure and powerful substances extracted from plants with steam. Undiluted, essential oils can burn your skin and may be toxic if taken internally.

BASIC RECIPE FOR HERBAL OIL, HOT METHOD

1. Combine the herbs and oil in a double boiler, cover the pan, and heat the mixture over low heat for 2 to 3 hours. Check periodically to be sure water in the bottom pan hasn't completely evaporated.
2. Strain the oil into a dark-colored bottle.

Storage. Up to one year in the refrigerator.

Use. As a massage oil for arthritis, muscle pain, or fatigue.

BASIC RECIPE FOR HERBAL OIL, COLD METHOD

1. Pack a clear glass jar with herbs, and cover them with oil. Cover the jar.
2. Put the jar in a sunny place for about two weeks. Give the jar a good shake once a day.
3. If the oil doesn't seem dark or aromatic enough after two weeks, add more herbs and repeat the process.
4. Strain the oil into a dark-colored bottle.

Storage. Up to one year in the refrigerator.

Use. As a massage oil for arthritis, muscle pain, or fatigue.

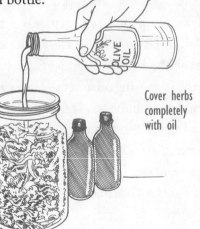

Cover herbs completely with oil

Ointments

Ointments are used to protect the skin from air and moisture. Non-penetrating, they form a barrier on the surface of the skin, shielding raw, irritated, or wounded areas while providing antibacterial and/or antifungal healing benefits.

BASIC RECIPE FOR AN OINTMENT, METHOD 1

1. Combine the tincture and lotion, and stir to mix well.
2. Pour into a small, clean jar.

Storage. Three to four months.

Uses. See below.

What You Need

½–1 teaspoon of tincture
1 ounce of commercial skin lotion

BASIC RECIPE FOR AN OINTMENT, METHOD 2

1. Combine the herbs and petroleum jelly in a double boiler, cover the pan, and heat over low heat for about 2 hours. Check the bottom pan periodically to be sure the water hasn't evaporated.
2. Remove from heat and cool slightly. But before the mixture cools and hardens (wear rubber gloves to keep from burning your hands), use a jelly bag or cloth to strain out the herbs and squeeze the jelly into a jar.

What You Need

2 ounces dried herb
16 ounces petroleum jelly

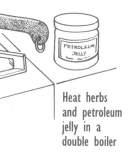

Heat herbs and petroleum jelly in a double boiler

Storage. Three to four months in the refrigerator.

Uses. Protect your skin from winter wind, soothe skin irritations such as diaper rash, or reduce the pain of hemorrhoids.

Salves

Although you can find a wide array of salves and creams at any health food store, you may enjoy making your own, tailored to your personal needs and aromatic preferences. Salves are thicker than ointments. Although recipes vary considerably, most of them call for beeswax, which you can find at health food stores in easy-to-measure 1-ounce cubes. Some recipes call for lanolin or glycerin, which can also be found in most stores that sell herbal products. You can make salves using either an infusion or a decoction (see Method 1 below) or dried herbs (see Method 2 on page 21).

BASIC RECIPE FOR A SALVE, METHOD I

1. Combine the infusion or decoction and oil in a saucepan, and heat over medium heat until any water evaporates. (If you have any doubt, remeasure to see that the total volume of the mix has been reduced by half.)
2. Melt the beeswax in a double boiler.
3. Stir the beeswax into the herb/oil mixture until it's of an even consistency. If you wish, add a few drops of essential oil of benzoin or myrrh to help preserve your salve. You can also add a few drops of your favorite essential oil to scent the mixture.
4. Pour the warm salve into a jar. When cooled, the salve will be the consistency of soft butter or petroleum jelly.

What You Need

- 1 part double-strength herbal infusion or decoction
- 1 part oil (a high-quality cooking oil, such as extra virgin olive, safflower, or grapeseed oil)
- 1 ounce beeswax
- A few drops of essential oil of benzoin or myrrh (optional)
- A few drops of fragrant essential oil (optional)

While still warm, pour the salve into a glass storage jar

BASIC RECIPE FOR A SALVE, METHOD 2

1. Melt the beeswax in a double boiler. Stir in the oil.
2. Shake in dried herbs until they are completely covered, but you don't see a lot of excess oil. Cook this mixture in a double boiler for 2 to 3 hours, checking occasionally to be sure there is enough water in the bottom pan.
3. If desired, stir in a few drops of essential oil of myrrh or benzoin as a preservative. You can also add a few drops of essential oil for fragrance.
4. Strain the mixture through a cloth into a jar.

Storage. Up to one year in the refrigerator.

Use. Massage sore backs or tired muscles, moisturize dry skin, or treat skin problems such as eczema, all depending on the herbs you choose to use in your salve.

What You Need

1 ounce beeswax
½ cup oil (a high-quality cooking oil, such as extra-virgin olive, safflower, or grapeseed oil
½–1 cup dried herbs
A few drops of essential oil of myrrh or benzoin (optional)
A few drops of fragrant essential oil (optional)

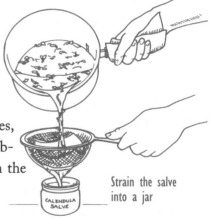

Strain the salve into a jar

Avoiding Mold

Mold can be a problem with herbal preparations, especially syrups, salves, and ointments. To prevent mold from forming, sterilize your containers. You can boil them for 10 minutes or use your oven or microwave (consult your owner's manual for directions on how to use your microwave for this purpose), but the easiest way is to use them right after they've been run through the dishwasher. It will also help if you keep the finished products refrigerated.

YOUR HERBAL MEDICINE CHEST

You've probably heard it said that medicine chests reveal quite a lot about their owners. As you develop your own herbal medicine chest, you'll no doubt customize it for you and your family. You won't need every herb described in this book and that's a good thing, since there are so many healing herbs you would never have room to grow or store them all. Obviously, you will choose the ones most appropriate for your home. No one in my family, for instance, has problems with motion sickness, but if we did, I would stock ginger well beyond what I need for cooking stir-fries and curry. If one of us suffered from migraines, I would plant several large clumps of feverfew. There are many problems, though, like bruises and sore throats — and aging — that are common to us all, so most basic medicine chests contain preparations to help heal burns and cuts, take the blue out of bruises, fight gingivitis, repel biting insects, ease indigestion, and banish headaches.

ESSENTIAL SUPPLIES TO HAVE ON HAND

In addition to herbs, you'll also want to stock up on some standard ingredients that you'll need for making your herbal preparations. These include **oil** (extra virgin olive, safflower, or grapeseed) for making herbal oil infusions and salves, **beeswax** for making salves, **honey or sugar** for flavoring bitter herbs and making syrups, **vodka** for tinctures, **wine** for tonics, **petroleum jelly** or **commercial skin lotion** for ointments, and **gelatin capsules** to make your own herb capsules. In addition, you will probably want to keep the following items on hand. You'll be able to find most of them in pharmacies, grocery stores, or health food stores.
Essential oils. Available commercially from many different kinds of plants, essential oils are highly concentrated oils that play a major role in aromatherapy. Used properly, they can be a luxurious treat. Put a few drops in a hot bath, or mix 5 or 10 drops with 1 ounce almond oil or other "carrier" oil, and use the mixture for massage. Essential oils may also be used as an ingredient in your homemade salves.
Safety first. Never take essential oils internally, as many are quite toxic. Some can irritate or burn your skin if used undiluted.

Gauze pads. Available in a variety of sizes, the smaller sizes are useful for protecting wounds after you've applied an herbal salve, for instance, and the larger ones make good compresses.

Gauze bandages. You'll find these, too, in a variety of sizes. The 2-inch width is good when you need to hold a compress in place.

Cotton balls. These are useful for applying herbal remedies to surface wounds or irritated skin.

Adhesive tape. You'll need this to hold gauze pads or compresses in place when it's inconvenient to wrap the area.

Tweezers. This multipurpose tool helps you extract splinters and ticks.

Eye cup. An eye cup is essential when you need to bathe irritated eyes with an herbal infusion or decoction. Be sure to strain the solution before use, to get rid of any pieces of herb that might get into your eye. To use, pour a few teaspoons of the medicine into the sterilized cup, place the cup against your eye, and, pressing the cup firmly against your eye, tilt your head back, blinking your eye several times.

> ## Storing Your Herbal Medicines
>
> Your herbal medicine chest may not be the one in your master bath. Most herbs and herbal preparations keep best in a cool dark place, and dried herbs should not be stored in areas of high humidity, like the kitchen and bathroom.

THE BASIC HERBS

The chart on the following pages includes 20 of the most useful herbs for treating the most common symptoms you and your family are likely to experience. You'll be able to see at a glance what herbs treat which symptoms, whether it's easier to grow or purchase the herbs, and advice on how to store them. You'll find more complete information about the herbs (including suggestions for dosage) in Chapter 3, "Essential Healing Herbs A to Z" (immediately following the chart), and about the symptoms in Chapter 5, "Symptoms and Remedies" (beginning on page 101).

A Basic Herbal Medicine Chest

HERB	USE IT FOR	HOW TO OBTAIN	HOW TO STORE
Aloe *Aloe vera*	Burns, bites, cuts, scrapes	Grow it year-round in containers.	Use fresh.
Calendula *Calendula officinalis*	Skin problems, ulcers	Buy as cream or grow it to make your own ointments or salves.	In refrigerator for up to three months.
Chaste tree *Vitex agnus-castus*	Menstrual cramps, menopause	Grow it for berries or buy berries to make a decoction.	Dry berries and store for up to one year.
Comfrey *Symphytum officinale*	Bruises, hemorrhoids	Grow it.	Dry leaves and store for up to one year.
Echinacea *Echinacea purpurea*	Preventing and treating colds and flu	Grow it to harvest roots, or purchase capsules or tincture.	Dry roots and store for up to one year.
Eucalyptus *Eucalyptus globulus*	Cold symptoms	Grow it, buy dried leaves, or buy essential oil.	Dry leaves and store for up to one year.
Garlic *Allium sativum*	Preventing cardiovascular problems, preventing and treating respiratory ailments, curing fungal infections, and treating acne	Grow it or buy it from your grocer.	In a cool, dry place for up to eight weeks.
Ginkgo *Ginkgo biloba*	Enhancing memory and alertness; preventing heart attack, stroke, and impotence	Buy capsules.	Consult label for freshness date.
Lavender *Lavandula* spp.	Headache, tense muscles; burns and sunburns; relaxant	Grow it or buy essential oil.	Keep bottle filled and check regularly for change in scent.
Lemon balm *Melissa officinalis*	Insomnia, anxiety, fever; skin injuries and cold sores; flavoring for other herb teas	Grow it.	Store dried leaves for up to one year.

HERB	USE IT FOR	HOW TO OBTAIN	HOW TO STORE
Licorice *Glycyrrhiza glabra*	Sore throats and coughs, gingivitis, canker sores; sweetening other herb teas	Buy fresh root or a tincture.	Store dried chopped roots for up to one year.
Milk thistle *Silybum marianum*	A healthy liver	Buy capsules or extract.	Consult label for freshness date.
Mint *Mentha x piperita* (peppermint); *M. spicata* (spearmint)	Heartburn, indigestion, nausea, bad breath; flavoring for other herb teas	Grow it.	Store dried leaves for up to one year.
Mountain mint *Pycnanthemum muticum*	Repelling insects	Grow it.	Use leaves fresh; store oil in a cool, dark place.
Psyllium *Plantago ovata*	Constipation	Buy it in prepared products.	Consult label for freshness date.
Red pepper *Capsicum* spp.	Muscle aches, arthritis	Grow it or buy capsules.	Dried peppers maintain heat indefinitely.
St.-John's-wort *Hypericum perforatum*	Depression, skin injuries	Buy capsules to treat depression; grow it for external use.	Consult label for freshness date; store dried leaves or flowers for up to one year.
Tea tree *Melaleuca alternifolia*	Skin injuries	Buy essential oil.	Consult label for directions.
Willow *Salix* spp.	Pain	Remove small amounts of bark from one side of a tree, or purchase bark.	Store dried bark for up to one year, tincture for up to two years.
Witch hazel *Hamamelis* spp.	Sunburn, insect bites, tired eyes, hemorrhoids	Buy the extract, or make a decoction from bark.	Store leaves and dried bark for up to one year.

Understanding Herbal Medicine Labels

Did you ever wonder why the labels on some herbal medicines are vague? For instance, you may see: "Suggested Use: Take 1 caplet one to three times daily with a full glass of water, preferably after a meal." Take it for what? Is it safe to take if I'm pregnant? What if I take a prescription medicine regularly? Are there any side effects?

When you buy commercial medicines, it's quite another story. The list of warnings is so long that it comes packed inside an otherwise extraneous box, in type so small you have to haul out a magnifying glass to read it. There's a reason for this. Congress passed federal drug laws to protect us from "snake-oil salesmen" and the horrors of untested drugs that in years past caused injury or death to unsuspecting users. Unfortunately, the laws have backfired when it comes to herbs.

Drug companies spend more than $200 million to bring one new medicine to market. They spend at least half that on testing, to prove that the drug really works and that it is safe. The companies are willing to foot these hefty bills because they can patent a new, unique medicine and reap all the profits for 17 years. But they won't make any money if they go through this process with herbs, because plants are already available to everyone at relatively little, or even no, cost. So herbs are considered foods, not drugs, and under current laws, the labels can't contain health claims. That doesn't mean they're not effective. Medicinal herbs have been used for centuries throughout the world, and a great deal of contemporary research continues to prove that they work.

Your own observations will soon prove how beneficial these natural healers can be. The labels will recommend a dose, based on a standardized minimal amount of active ingredients. (When you purchase herbs, look for the words "standardized" or "standardized formula" on the label.) Don't take more than the recommended amount. Remember: If a little of something is good, a lot is not always better.

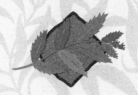

CHAPTER 3

ESSENTIAL
Healing Herbs
A *to* Z

Many of the plants we now take for granted in our gardens and landscapes — from roses and willow trees to carrots and garlic — were first recognized as herbs. Even plants we regard as weeds, such as the common mullein *(Verbascum thapsus)*, were brought to this continent by the early European settlers as treasured herbs. With so many rich and varied possibilities, you're not alone if you wonder which herbs are best to use for which problems. The herbs in this chapter are those most frequently used today, and recent research backs their power and safety. You can grow most of them in gardens throughout the United States, or obtain them readily in health food stores or even supermarkets.

ALOE *Aloe vera*

Parts used: Gel from inside the leaves

Even if you think of yourself as a complete herbal novice, if you have this fleshy succulent on your kitchen windowsill, you are already familiar with one of the world's most ancient, time-honored, and dependable herbal remedies. If you burn a finger or get careless with a paring knife, simply break off a leaf. The soothing antibacterial and antifungal gel inside the leaf not only gives prompt pain relief but speeds healing as well. Though you can buy many excellent commercial preparations containing aloe — including skin lotions and shampoos — keep the real thing on hand for full-powered home healing.

Aloe

EXTERNAL USE

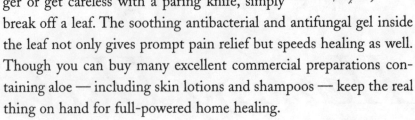

Skin injuries. In an emergency, quickly cut off part of a leaf and rub the exposed gel against your skin. If the situation requires less immediate attention — for instance, if you've spent too much time in the sun without your sunscreen — cut off part of a leaf and, using a small knife, peel off the thin skin. Squeeze the gel into a jar and cool it in the refrigerator for added relief, but use it within hours, as it does not keep.

Other uses. Applied the same way as for other skin injuries, aloe is helpful for insect bites, acne, shingles, eczema, wrinkles, stretch marks, and most problems involving dry itchy skin. Overexposed to the winter elements? Aloe in your first-aid kit may help with frostbite, since there is evidence that it stimulates blood circulation.

Safety First. While aloe vera is completely safe when used externally, never use aloe internally. In health food stores you may see a laxative labeled "aloe", but it is made from plant cells found just beneath the outer covering of the leaf, not the gel. Even when professionally prepared, it can cause painful cramps.

IN THE GARDEN

With its plump, slick, yellow-banded leaves, aloe is an easy-to-recognize plant. Most of us have to grow it indoors, as it's a tropical plant and won't tolerate temperatures below 40°F. While aloe is undemanding, generous watering will keep the leaves fat and gel-filled. If you put it outside in summer, give it light shade so the hot sun doesn't shrivel the leaves. The plant will make dozens of little offsets that you can dig out to share with friends. For variety, group aloe in a container with other low-care succulents. The mature plant sends up a spike hung with yellow-orange, tubular flowers.

ANGELICA *Angelica archangelica*
Parts used: Leaves, seeds, and roots

Tradition says this towering European perennial got its name in the mid-1600s, when a monk dreamed that an angel told him the herb would cure bubonic plague. Often a symbol of innocence — women in the Middle Ages planted it around their homes to show that they weren't witches — it's also an ingredient in alcoholic beverages, including Benedictine and gin.

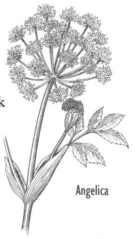

Angelica

Two other species are sometimes used for medicine: *Angelica sinensis,* from China, often called dong quai, and an American native, *A. atropurpurea.* Angelica is useful as a treatment for indigestion. Like many herbs that relax uterine muscles, angelica also relaxes the digestive system.

INTERNAL USES

Heartburn and indigestion. Make an infusion with 1 teaspoon of dried herb or seeds in 1 cup of water, or a decoction using 1 to 3 teaspoons of the dried root in 1 cup of water. Drink up to two cups a day.
Increased libido. Dong quai is a big seller in health food stores. Its reputation as a female tonic and aphrodisiac may explain its widespread popularity. (Traditionally, it is also used to regulate menstrual periods and reduce their unpleasant symptoms.) If you make your own decoction, use 1 to 3 teaspoons of dried root per cup of water.
Other uses. Used for thousands of years for respiratory problems, angelica relaxes the windpipe, making it soothing for cold, flu, or bronchitis. Research suggests that it may also ease the pain of arthritis. Use either an infusion or a decoction as described above.

An Old-Fashioned Treat

Pick fresh stems of angelica and cook them as you would asparagus. Or, turn this sweet, licorice-flavored herb into an old-fashioned confection. Cut fresh, second-year stems short enough to fit in a cooking pan. Blanch them for 2 minutes, peel them, and cut them into 2-inch pieces. Simmer for 20 minutes in a syrup of equal parts sugar and water. Drain off the syrup, place the stems and syrup in a covered container, and refrigerate. After three or four days, reheat the angelica in the syrup for about 20 minutes. Drain off any remaining syrup and dry the stems on waxed paper.

The stalks are usually ground up and used as a flavoring in cakes and other desserts.

Safety first. The fresh root is phototoxic, meaning that some people who consume a lot of angelica develop a supersensitivity to sunlight. Be sure to dry it thoroughly. Angelica should not be used during pregnancy without consulting a physician.

IN THE GARDEN

You won't be able to hide this tall, stately plant, which has been described as a 4-foot-tall carrot, so you might as well make it the centerpiece of a shady herb garden. The stems are bold and the leaves have three parts. The midsummer flowers are greenish white umbels, sometimes 6 inches across, and have a honeylike fragrance. Angelica is a monocarp, which means that once it flowers and produces seeds, it dies. But you can keep it going from year to year if you remove the flowerheads and don't ever let it go to seed. If you do let it produce seeds, however, it tends to self-sow, giving you an ongoing supply of the plant in your garden. Southern gardeners find that angelica does not like their hot summers. The fresh roots are poisonous, so take care to dry them thoroughly before using. Dry for at least two months, or until the roots break easily. *Zones 4–7.*

BLACK COHOSH *Cimicifuga racemosa*
Parts used: Roots and rhizomes

I enjoy growing native plants for many reasons, but especially for the folk wisdom associated with them. Most of the common names for this plant have to do with its roots: They're black and gnarly (*cohosh* is an Indian word for "rough") and were used to treat

Black Cohosh

rattlesnake bites, so it's not surprising to learn that another of its common names is snakeroot. Native Americans also used black cohosh to treat menstrual discomfort, and that's how most herbalists use it today. All evidence shows that it really works, although it may have some side effects, and studies on its long-term safety are few.

INTERNAL USE

Menstrual discomfort. Simmer ½ teaspoon of powdered root in 1 cup of water, covered, for 15 minutes, and flavor with lemon and honey. Take no more than a cup a day, in small doses.

Safety first. Some herbalists feel that black cohosh is extremely safe; others say it can have side effects, such as dizziness, nausea, and headaches. If you experience side effects, discontinue use. Do not use black cohosh during pregnancy or while breastfeeding.

IN THE GARDEN

This giant perennial is also called fairy candles, for the shape of its white flower spikes. It can reach 8 feet tall when it blooms. In midsummer the flowers start out as tiny white button buds, opening from the bottom up into fragrant little bottle brushes. The lacy leaves look like astilbe foliage. A woodland native, it prefers shade. *Zones 3–7.*

CALENDULA *Calendula officinalis*
Parts used: Flowers, harvested when newly opened

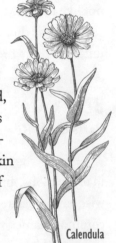

Calendula

Pot marigold is another name for this annual. Botanically, it isn't related to the common marigold, *Tagetes,* but the golden yellow color of the flower is similar. (Don't substitute common marigold as a medicinal herb.) Calendula is good for all kinds of skin problems, including acne and the speedy healing of wounds and burns. It combats bacteria, fungus infections, viruses, and inflammation.

INTERNAL USE

Ulcers. James Duke, author of *The Green Pharmacy,* says calendula's power against inflammation works in the stomach as well as on the skin. He makes a tea with 2 teaspoons of calendula flowers per 1 cup of water, and gives it zip with a bit of lemon juice or lemon balm. Others suggest combining calendula, meadowsweet, and chamomile.

Acne. Use a calendula cream to cleanse your face.

Dry skin, rashes, burns, bruises, and fungal infections. You can find calendula cream at health food stores, or make your own ointment or salve following the standard recipes described on pages 19–21.

Cuts. Make an infusion using 2 to 3 teaspoons of dried herbs to 1 cup of water, and apply it with a compress. Or make a tincture and apply it directly to the cut with a cotton ball.

Insect bites and stings. Treat as you would burns or cuts, or simply grab some fresh flowers from the garden and rub them directly on the bite.

Other uses. Steep 2 teaspoons of dried flower petals in 1 cup of water, strain, and use as a mouthwash or gargle for a sore throat, tonsillitis, and canker sores in your mouth.

IN THE GARDEN

Pot marigold flowers range from yellow to orange, with single or double petals. They bloom six weeks after you plant the seeds, and continue well into early winter. Up to 2 feet tall, they make a cheerful edge for a border, but will need some shade in the South. If you harvest their heads regularly, you will encourage even more flowers.

CATNIP *Nepeta cataria*

Parts used: Flowering tops and, less powerfully, leaves

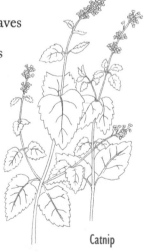

Most of us are familiar with the cartoon capers of catnip-inebriated felines, and almost every pet store offers an array of clever catnip kitten toys. This herb drives most cats absolutely bonkers. Oddly enough, it has an opposite, calming effect on humans.

The plant's species name will help you remember another potential use: preventing cataracts, a clouding of the eye that will eventually affect about half of us who live past the age of 75.

Catnip

Mild sedative. To relax before bedtime or after a hard day at the office, brew 2 teaspoons of the dried herb in 1 cup of hot water.

Stomach soother. Like other members of the mint family, catnip relaxes the muscles of the digestive system and may ease menstrual cramps, too. Brew 2 teaspoons of the dried herb in 1 cup of water.

Cataract prevention. If you are diabetic, you are at higher risk for cataracts and might want to include a catnip infusion in your nightly regimen. Brew 2 teaspoons of the dried herb in 1 cup of hot water.

IN THE GARDEN

This 3-foot-tall perennial has small, understated white or purple flowers that bloom on spikes in midsummer. Its fuzzy gray leaves will set off your greener herbs. Catnip is at its best in the slightly sandy soil and full sun of a traditional herb bed. It is sometimes mistakenly called catmint, which is a different, more ornamental species (*N. mussinii*). Bruising the leaves of catnip releases its cat-calling aroma. Some gardeners say this won't happen if you start it from seed, but cats will find it anyway, so don't put it near delicate plants that could be crushed in the feline frenzy. *Zones 3–9.*

CHAMOMILE *Matricaria chamomilla, Chamaemelum nobile*

Parts used: Flower heads, fresh or dried

Even if you are just beginning to explore the world of herbs, you're probably already familiar with chamomile, a favorite for commercial bedtime teas. And if you remember your Beatrix Potter, you may recall Mother Rabbit calling for Peter Rabbit to fetch some more chamomile. Peter ignores her and gets into his usual mischief, but it's hard to get into trouble growing or using this charming, sweet-scented herb.

German Chamomile

The two different chamomiles — German or Hungarian chamomile *(Matricaria chamomilla)* and Roman chamomile *(Chamaemelum nobile)* — are distant cousins in the aster family, both native to Europe. Even though these plants aren't closely related, our ancestors used them for similar purposes — for digestive problems and for skin irritations. The German variety is the one you're more likely to find in commercial American herbal products.

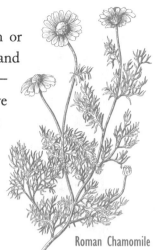

Roman Chamomile

Relaxant. As a sleep inducer, chamomile is considered safe enough for children. (With a little milk, it might make a nice companion to those Peter Rabbit stories.) It appears to work by depressing the central nervous system. Because it is a relaxant, it may alleviate tension headaches. Make an infusion using 1 teaspoon of the dried herb in 1 cup of water.

Digestion. Chamomile has been used for 2,000 years to soothe the digestive system — offering relief from irritable bowel syndrome, bloating, and ulcers. It contains a strong antispasmodic, which relaxes the digestive tract. Make an infusion using 1 teaspoon of the dried herb in 1 cup of water.

Menstrual cramps. Those same antispasmodic properties also help relieve painful menstrual cramps. Make an infusion using 1 teaspoon of the dried herb in 1 cup of water.

EXTERNAL USES

Skin irritations. Make a chamomile infusion using 1 heaping tablespoon of the dried herb in 1 cup of water and apply as a compress to bites, stings, burns, tired eyes, and nipples irritated by nursing.

IN THE GARDEN

German chamomile is a hardy annual, which may reseed and appear the following year if it's planted in a sunny spot and receives regular watering. The ferny foliage makes a pleasing contrast to heavier-leaved herbs like basil, and the cheerful, daisylike flowers last from early summer into autumn. Chamomile can range anywhere from 6 inches to 2 feet tall. *Herbal Renaissance* author Steven Foster says that in Boulder, Colorado, home of Celestial Seasonings teas, it pops up along roads and in sidewalk cracks. In many parts of the Northeast, it's a common sight along the edges of fields and roadways.

The perennial, Roman chamomile, has coarser leaves, tends to creep, and is tough enough to walk on. Plant it among flagstones and enjoy its sweet aroma as you saunter down the path.

CHASTE TREE *Vitex agnus-castus*
Parts used: Dried fruit

Chaste trees gets its name because of the ancient use of its seeds as an antiaphrodisiac. They were ground up and used as a seasoning in monasteries, and came to be called monk's pepper. Today herbalists still use the seeds to treat the reproductive system.

Chaste
Tree

INTERNAL USES
Menopausal symptoms. No one has identified which compounds make them work, but chaste tree berries regulate hormones. The result, for some women, is a reduction in uncomfortable symptoms such as hot flashes. The recommended dose is 20 to 40 mg a day — about ⅛ teaspoon of the powdered fruits.

Premenstrual syndrome. A British study found a 60 percent reduction in such symptoms as nervous tension and mood changes among women who took chaste berry capsules. Follow dosage instructions on purchased standardized formula.

Other uses. The dried fruit of chaste tree seems to reduce premenstrual water retention and increase milk production in nursing mothers. Follow instructions on purchased standardized formula.

IN THE GARDEN

The deliciously pungent foliage of chaste tree looks suspiciously like marijuana, so some of your neighbors may raise their eyebrows if you plant a chaste tree in your front yard. It is naturally shrubby, and grows 9 to 17 feet tall, but you can prune it into a small tree. Severe pruning of all its small branches — called pollarding — makes it bloom more heavily. Although the chaste tree also grows naturally in West Asia, the narrow gray leaves are very similar to those of other plants that grow in the Mediterranean region. In midsummer it makes an absolute spectacle of itself, erupting with spikes of bright lavender flowers. The berries, about the size of mustard seeds, are briefly pink, then they dry and turn gray, so they're more aptly described as seeds. Chaste tree is quite simple to grow. The seeds germinate easily and it will self-sow in a fertile garden. In Zone 6, it may sometimes get zapped by cold temperatures, but it should regrow from the roots if you prune it back to about 1 foot tall in the spring. In these cooler areas it will remain a shrub, growing only 3 to 4 feet tall. *Zones 7–9.*

More Relief for Menopausal Symptoms

Red clover (*Trifolium pratense*) will enrich your garden when you grow it in the off-season and then plow it under. Called a cover crop, or green manure, it adds nitrogen to your soil. But red clover might make you more healthy, too. It contains a number of antitumor chemicals, and others that act like estrogen, the female hormone. This means that along with chaste tree, it could help ease symptoms of menopause. The red ball flowers are edible and make a sweet-tasting drink. Use an infusion made with up to 3 teaspoons of the dried flowers in 1 cup of water.

Red Clover

ECHINACEA *Echinacea angustifolia,*
E. purpurea

Parts used: Roots, harvested in their second
year, and flowers

Also called purple coneflower, this herb has
absolutely everything going for it. Its color and
shape work well in every garden, and it's irresistible to
butterflies. It was a favorite medicinal plant of the Plains
Indians, and today much scientific evidence indicates that
it can keep our immune systems in tip-top shape. Researchers are also
studying echinacea to see if it is among the herbs that slow the aging
process. It has received so much good press recently that people in the
United States buy more echinacea than any other herb.

There are several echinacea species, all native to the central
United States and varying only slightly in appearance, but most of the
echinacea sold as capsules and extracts is made from *Echinacea purpurea.* Varro Tyler, author of *The Honest Herbal,* believes that the
extract is more effective than capsules, although it is somewhat
expensive. Echinacea will make your tongue tingle, but that's normal,
and if you've made your own decoction, the tingle may serve as a sign
that the dose is strong enough.

INTERNAL USE

Preventing colds and flu. Studies show that people who take echinacea have fewer, milder colds. It appears to work by both strengthen-
ing the immune system and fighting viruses. Some herbalists feel that
people who are prone to getting a lot of colds should take echinacea
regularly as a preventive. Others recommend that you use a decoction
made from 2 teaspoons of dried root per 1 cup of water at the first sign
of a cold, or when you think you've been exposed to a virus. Echinacea
makes an effective mouthwash and gargle for sore throats and tonsili-
tis, although it tends to numb the mouth.

Yeast infections. In the past couple of decades, vaginal yeast infections have become more common among American women. One

reason is that we use too many antibiotics, which tend to knock out our natural defenses against this fungus. Taking an echinacea decoction (2 teaspoons of dried root in 1 cup of water) for a week or so can help.

Other uses. Herbalists often use echinacea to treat chronic fatigue syndrome. If you use it as a mouthwash, its antibacterial properties can help prevent gingivitis.

IN THE GARDEN

Coneflowers are beautiful in any type of natural planting, such as meadows and butterfly gardens. The flowers of most species, including *E. angustifolia* and *E. purpurea,* are pink to purple, but *E. paradoxa* is yellow, and there are some white cultivars. *E. pallida* has dramatically drooping petals. All of them take full sun except *E. purpurea,* a native of the open woods that can tolerate some light shade. *E. purpurea* generally grows about 4 feet tall; some of the other species are a bit shorter. The common name comes from the prickly upright cone in the center, which remains eye-catching in the autumn garden long after the petals have fallen. Coneflowers are drought-tolerant but can be magnets for Japanese beetles. *Zones 3–8.*

Don't Collect Herbs from the Wild

We're loving some herbs to death. There are too few herb farmers growing them for commercial purposes, and too many people willing to collect them for quick cash; American ginseng, goldenseal, and echinacea are disappearing from the fields and forests where they grow naturally. Don't add to the problem by collecting any herbs that are not growing on your own land.

Another reason not to collect in the wild is that you don't know whether the plants have been treated with pesticides. And, of course, never use any herb if you're not 100 percent sure about what it is.

Making Flu Flee

Along with echinacea, another flu-fighting herb is elderberry. Most of us have heard of the American native shrub elderberry (*Sambucus canadensis*) as the source of elderberry wine. A European species (*S. nigra*) was used as a laxative for hundreds of years, but it's now considered too strong. You should avoid all unripe parts of elderberries (including leaf buds, green berries, and green shoots), and some herbalists feel that the American species is more toxic when unripe. In the 1980s, Israeli researchers found a substance in the leaves of *S. nigra* that cures some strains of flu by preventing the viruses from invading the respiratory system. It is now available in this country under the brand name Sambucol.

EVENING PRIMROSE *Oenothera biennis*

Parts used: Seeds, for the extraction of oil

This native biennial was once considered a cure-all, but is now viewed with some skepticism in the United States. The oil that's processed from its tiny seeds is rich in a substance called gamma-linolenic acid (GLA), which addresses a number of seemingly unrelated problems that occur when our bodies don't have enough essential fatty acids. These include premenstrual syndrome and the breast pain that often accompanies it, eczema, the effects of alcoholism, diabetes, and possibly some forms of cancer.

Evening
Primrose

INTERNAL USE

Premenstrual syndrome. Native American women used evening primrose for centuries. Today, herbalists say you need to buy capsules of the processed oil to get real medicinal benefits. The usual recommended dose is three to six capsules a day.

Weight loss. James Duke writes in *The Green Pharmacy* that the tryptophan in evening primrose seed can make you feel more satisfied after a meal. If you can't get seeds, take ½ teaspoon of oil three times a day.

Safety first. *Don't use evening primrose oil if you have epilepsy.*

IN THE GARDEN

Because it can be somewhat invasive, many people consider the evening primrose a weed, but I can't resist letting *O. biennis* stay in just a few places where it pops up. The first year it's a flat rosette, then during its second year it develops 3- to 8-foot stems with branches that are loaded with buds. Every evening it opens pale yellow, four-petaled flowers that seem to glow in the dusk. You can restrain its self-sowing propensity by removing some of the seedpods that start forming after each flower's one night of glory. The pods are crammed with seeds, each not much bigger than a grain of salt.

Beautiful Biennial

Although you may have to buy a commercial product to obtain the evening primrose's medicinal benefits, the plant itself has uses. All parts are edible — the leaves in salads, the roots as a boiled vegetable, and the seeds on bread, like poppy seed.

FENNEL *Foeniculum vulgare*
Parts used: Seeds and, less powerfully, leaves

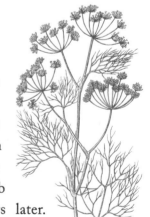

Fennel

Fennel is the marathon herb — that's what the ancient Greeks called it. Marathon was a town near Athens where fennel grew naturally. When the Athenians fought a victorious battle in Marathon in 490 B.C., they sent a runner to Athens with the big news, and the association of the town's famous herb with this joyous run still lingers, 2,500 years later. Hildegard of Bingen, a Benedictine abbess who wrote a famous herbal in the 12th century, said it was good for the health of our hearts, made us happy, and stopped body odor.

Indigestion. Like its close relatives anise, caraway, and dill, fennel will calm a jittery or gassy stomach. Simmer 1 or 2 teaspoons of crushed seeds in 1 cup of water.

Menstrual discomfort. Fennel may help with cramps, fluid retention, and premenstrual syndrome. Simmer 1 or 2 teaspoons of crushed seeds in 1 cup of water.

Other uses. Fennel will sweeten bad breath and may ease asthma symptoms. Simmer 1 or 2 teaspoons of crushed seeds in 1 cup of water.

Safety first. Michael and Janet Weiner, authors of Herbs That Heal, *say fresh fennel seeds may be irritating. They recommend storing them for a year before crushing them to make decoctions for internal use. Others say that chewing a tiny pinch of seeds is usually quite safe.*

Relaxant. A fennel bath can relax tired muscles and aching joints. Tie a small handful of whole seeds and dried leaves in cheesecloth and run your bathwater over it. Fennel will also help reduce body odor.

Eyewash. A traditional use of fennel is to soothe the eyes. Make a decoction using ½ teaspoon of crushed whole seeds in 1 cup of water. Strain carefully before using. Dilute if you experience any discomfort. Apply the wash from an eyecup, available at pharmacies.

Resembling a 7-foot dill plant — and smelling a bit like it, too — feathery fennel sways in the breeze and looks downright exotic. Although the seeds of all fennel varieties may be used medicinally, bronze fennel (*F. vulgare* 'Purpureum') is the more ornamental species, and Florence fennel *(F. vulgare* var. *azoricum)* is grown for the bulb so valued in cooking. Fennel can be invasive, but if you control it by snipping off the flat-topped flower heads, you won't get any of the little ribbed, football-shaped seeds that contain the most potent medicine. One solution is to watch for the seeds to start forming and tie a bag around the head to catch them as they fall. *Zones 5–9.*

FEVERFEW *Tanacetum parthenium*

Parts used: Leaves and flowering tops

John Gerard, in his 17th-century herbal, was only somewhat off base when he recommended feverfew for "them that are giddie in the head." Fifty years later, Nicholas Culpeper advised for a headache "the herb being bruised and applied to the crown of the head." Western medicine realized its potential for treating migraines less than 30 years ago.

Feverfew

You may think that feverfew got its name because the ancients used it to lower elevated body temperature. But Michael Castleman, author of *The Healing Herbs,* says the plant's early uses were for menstrual and birth-related problems. The common name, he says, derives from "featherfoil," describing its foliage.

INTERNAL USE

Migraine headaches. If you're among the one-in-eight Americans who get knocked off their feet by these recurring, blinding pains, you may find relief in simply chewing the fresh or dried leaves of feverfew. Unfortunately, the leaves taste bitter and cause mouth sores in about 12 percent of people who try them. If you can't stand the taste, make an infusion and add honey. Steep 1 teaspoon of dried herb in 1 cup of water. Or, purchase tablets or capsules; follow label directions for use.

Other uses. A close relative of chamomile, feverfew can be similarly soothing for an upset stomach.

IN THE GARDEN

Feverfew's flowers are almost dead ringers for Roman chamomile's, but the plant grows upright instead of sprawling. Daisylike flowers start appearing midsummer on this perennial, which grows to about 2 feet tall. Give it full sun and well-drained soil. Bees dislike it, which is great if you are allergic to their sting, but don't plant it near any crop plants that depend on bees for pollination. *Zones 5–7.*

GARLIC *Allium sativum*

Parts used: Bulb

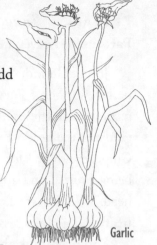

Garlic

You've got to hand it to a plant that will add zip to your pizza, cure acne, repel aphids, keep away vampires, and possibly prevent heart disease and some forms of cancer. It is said that the Egyptians gave garlic to the slaves who built the pyramids, and King Tut had some in his tomb. This member of the lily family is a great culinary condiment all over the world, but cooking breaks down its most powerful chemicals. Toss it into your recipes at the last minute, or eat it raw to take advantage of garlic's medicinal benefits.

INTERNAL USES

Cardiovascular disease prevention. Evidence is strong for garlic's ability to lower cholesterol (onions are almost as good) and high blood pressure, and to prevent clots that can cause heart attacks. You need to chew at least 3 to 10 cloves a day to reap this benefit.

You may find drinking garlic easier than eating it. Make a maceration (a cold infusion) of 6 crushed cloves in 1 cup of water. Let it steep 6 hours. A tincture made with ¼ cup of cloves in 1 cup of brandy may be more tasty; take up to 3 tablespoons a day of this tincture.

Cold and flu prevention. Garlic contains a powerful antibiotic that helps ward off respiratory infections, including bronchitis. Use as described above.

Diabetes. Garlic, as well as onions, seems to help lower blood sugar.

Other uses. Garlic protects the liver from lead poisoning and other toxins, may slow aging, and kills intestinal parasites. It also appears to keep certain cancer cells from forming.

EXTERNAL USES

Fungal infections. For problems like athlete's foot, crush 3 or 4 cloves of garlic with a garlic press and dab the problem area with a cotton ball.

Acne. For its antiseptic and antibacterial properties, rub a garlic clove directly on pimples. (You might not want to do this right before a big date!)

Earache. If you are sure that the eardrum is not punctured, you can put a few drops of garlic oil directly in the ear. The garlic provides both antiseptic and antibacterial benefits.

Bites and stings. To reduce the pain from bites and stings, make a garlic poultice by mashing 1 or 2 cloves of raw garlic and applying it directly to the affected area.

IN THE GARDEN

Garlic isn't a beautiful plant, but with its medicinal résumé, it doesn't need to be. It forms clumps of pungent leaves that look like floppy cornstalks, only they're 2 feet tall. All it asks of you is deep, rich, well-drained soil and a lot of sun. Start plants from cloves in either spring or fall, and keep the white flower clusters snipped off so the bulbs keep getting bigger until you harvest them — in midsummer for fall-planted bulbs, in fall for those you planted in spring. *Zones 5–9.*

Fangs a Lot!

Cabbage moths, Japanese beetles, and aphids apparently don't like garlic any more than Count Dracula did. Plant garlic, or another *Allium*, near cabbages or roses to discourage aphids and Japanese beetles, both of which adore these plants. If this fails, crush a dozen garlic cloves in a pint of water, and spritz the plants as needed to keep pests at bay.

GINGER *Zingiber officinale*
Parts used: Root

After a hearty meal, the ancient Greeks gave digestion a boost with a ginger sandwich, consisting of a piece of gingerroot wrapped in bread. This custom is thought to be a precursor to our gingerbread. Ginger is a necessity to keep on hand if members of your household have problems with motion sickness.

Ginger

Store gingerroot in a jar of sherry in the refrigerator. Slice what you need and peel before grating.

INTERNAL USES

Motion sickness. Ginger packs a double whammy by working against both dizziness and nausea. You can make a decoction with 3 teaspoons of finely grated fresh gingerroot to 1 cup of water, although purchased capsules may be handier for travelers. Even drinking ginger ale (if it contains real ginger) can calm a roiling tummy. You can suck on crystallized ginger, too.

Digestive problems. A ginger decoction (2 teaspoons of finely grated fresh gingerroot to 1 cup of water) aids digestion and, because it reduces stomach juices, may prevent ulcers.

Heart disease and stroke. Ginger helps keep blood from clotting and lowers cholesterol. Drink one or two cups of a ginger decoction a day.

Colds, sinusitis, viruses, and fever. Ginger contains several compounds with power against cold viruses, and others that ease symptoms such as fever and cough. Use as described above.

EXTERNAL USES

Toothache. Add a small amount of water to powdered ginger and use a cotton swab to apply it to the painful area, or press a cut section of fresh root to the area.

IN THE GARDEN

Ginger is a tropical perennial, so you will need a greenhouse to grow it if you live north of Zone 9. Ginger grows from the eye of the root, like a potato. Look for a green one in an Asian market and plant it 3 inches deep. It will develop a 3-foot stem with lance-shaped leaves and a single large yellow and purple flower. You will be able to harvest a much larger root after about nine months; use most of it and replant the rest to keep your ginger crop going. *Zones 10–11.*

GINKGO *Ginkgo biloba*

Parts used: Leaves

This Asian tree, sometimes called maidenhair, is one of the oldest on the planet. But the Western world didn't get excited about its health benefits until about two decades ago. Today it's the third most popular herb in the United States, right behind echinacea and garlic.

Ginkgo

INTERNAL USES

Memory retention. As we get older, many body processes become sluggish. For example, platelet activation factor (PAF) can slow blood flow to our brain, so our memory is no longer as sharp as it was. Ginkgo not only interferes with this slowdown but has even been shown to reverse the process in older people. If you want to take ginkgo, you will need to buy a commercial product. Look for tablets made from an extract of the leaves and follow label directions.

Heart attack and stroke. Ginkgo prevents stroke in the same way that it improves memory: by keeping open the blood vessels in the brain. It prevents heart attack by improving blood flow to that all-important muscle. Purchase tablets and follow label directions.

Impotence. An erection is another body function that depends on vigorous blood circulation. Clinical trials have shown that ginkgo can help some men when poor blood circulation is the cause of their impotence.

Safety first. Because you'll want to take ginkgo on a long-term basis, you should talk to your doctor about it. And remember that memory loss may be a sign of other health problems that require medical attention.

Other uses. As ginkgo stimulates blood flow, it may also dispel fatigue and depression.

IN THE GARDEN

You can't grow enough ginkgo to use as medicine, and harvesting the leaves would be a stretch, so to speak, since the tree can grow to be 100 feet tall. Even if you can't harvest your own ginkgo, consider one of these ancient trees for your landscape. The cultivar 'Autumn Gold' grows only 50 feet tall, and another, 'Princeton Sentry', is narrower than the species. Turning an intense yellow in fall, the fan-shaped leaves impart a sense of the Orient. Choose a male tree, though. The seeds inside the female fruits are edible, but the fruits themselves, which drop in staggering numbers in late summer, have an extremely nauseating smell. *Zones 5–9.*

GINSENG *Panax quinquefolius, P. ginseng, Eleutherococcus senticosus*
Parts used: Root

American Ginseng

Even though Siberian ginseng *(Eleutherococcus sen- ticosus)* isn't related to American ginseng *(Panax quin- quefolius)* and Korean ginseng *(P. ginseng),* they all have similar powers: enhanced performance and protection from stress. For the Chinese, Korean ginseng is full of magic. They once believed that it grew where lightning struck the ground. Because the roots have a vaguely human shape, they called it *jen shen* ("man root"). By the 1700s, the Chinese valued ginseng so highly as a tonic and aphrodisiac that they had just about wiped it out, but then Canadian Jesuits began shipping them the American species. Korean ginseng is the most thoroughly studied and the most expensive; less costly Siberian ginseng is more likely to be found in commercial products in the U.S. Siberian ginseng is less likely than the other species to have the undesirable side effect of insomnia.

Korean Ginseng

INTERNAL USES
Stimulating the immune system. Herbalists call plants like ginseng "adaptogenic," which means that they normalize body functions, for instance, lowering high blood pressure or raising low blood pressure to

normal. That seems pretty sweeping, but ginseng keeps us in general good health by bolstering our body's immune system. By custom, the Chinese simply chew on the root. You can decoct 2 slices or ½ teaspoon of dried root powder in 1 cup of hot water, and drink two cups a day. Commercial ginseng products are often adulterated; one study found that a quarter of ginseng products didn't contain any of the substance at all! To

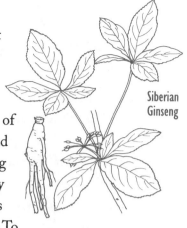

Siberian Ginseng

ensure that you are purchasing a high-quality product, look for "standardized herbal extract" on the label. Herbalists consider 250 mg an effective daily dose. Some labels specify that the capsules are made from six-year-old roots, helping to assure you of their potency.

Counteracting fatigue and enhancing performance. Ginseng increases the ability to handle mental and emotional stress, hunger, and temperature extremes. It improves coordination, concentration, and memory, and boosts energy. Decoct 2 slices or ½ teaspoon of dried root powder in 1 cup of hot water.

Other uses. Ginseng may reduce blood sugar, protect the liver against toxins, dispel depression, and protect cancer patients against radiation. Prepare a decoction as described above.

Safety first. Many herbalists suggest taking ginseng for only a month, then stopping for two or three months before using it again. Use cautiously if you have high blood pressure. Avoid using during pregnancy.

IN THE GARDEN

Ginseng is a perennial ground cover, related to ivy. For its first two years, its leaves have three parts, like a strawberry's. After that, the plant starts developing its characteristic five-part leaves. The tiny greenish white flowers bloom in June or July, then give way to bright red berries. Growing your own ginseng will not bring instant gratification, since the seeds can take a year to germinate, and the root will not have full medicinal potency for six years.

GOLDENSEAL *Hydrastis canadensis*

Parts used: Rhizome and roots, dried and powdered

When I asked my brother-in-law, who owns a successful health food store, how I could make a living at my 6-acre weekend property, he replied: "Become a goldenseal farmer." He knows how popular this herb has become — number four on the herbal hit parade.

Goldenseal

Native Americans used the root as a dye, to repel insects, to treat skin diseases, and as an eyewash. In the late '70s, a popular mystery writer advanced the notion — untrue — that it would prevent opiates from being detected in urine. Although some herbalists question its ability to stimulate the immune system, it still gets high marks for its antibacterial qualities.

Safety first: Do not use if you're pregnant or if you have high blood pressure.

INTERNAL USES

Stimulating the immune system. This use is now controversial, but it still has supporters. They say it works by stimulating our white blood cells, which defend us against bacteria, viruses, and fungi. Use ½ to 1 teaspoon of powdered root to make 1 cup of decoction, and drink up to two cups a day. Add honey to mask its bitter taste.

Diarrhea. Goldenseal's ability to wipe out microorganisms makes it useful to treat diarrhea, particularly the variety we can pick up when we travel and encounter bacteria that our systems aren't accustomed to. Buy tablets and follow label instructions.

Sinus problems and earache. Goldenseal's antibiotic properties work on sinus infections, at the same time relieving pressure on the middle ear. Buy tablets and follow label directions.

EXTERNAL USE

Skin injuries and infections. Put goldenseal's antiseptic properties into action when you have a cut, burn, fungal infection, or sty (an infection that shows as a reddened bump on an eyelid). Since you won't swallow the preparation, you can make a strong decoction with 3 or more teaspoons of dried root in 1 cup of water.

Sore throats and canker sores. Goldenseal is an antiseptic and astringent, so you can put it to work against mouth and throat discomfort by using it as a gargle. Make a decoction with 1 teaspoon of dried root in 1 cup of water. It's bitter, so have some flavorings on hand.

IN THE GARDEN

Goldenseal is a perennial in the buttercup family that's considered hard to grow. And, it's no great beauty. It sends up a foot-tall hairy, purplish stem, which has two large, lobed leaves. The flowers, which are balls of greenish-white stamens without any petals, bloom in midspring for a week or less; it then bears raspberry-like fruits in midsummer. You'll need a five-year-old root to use as a medicine, so if you do grow goldenseal, start with two-year-old root pieces and plant them in deep shade, since goldenseal is a native woodland plant. The stem dies back every year, leaving a scar, so you can count the stem scars to determine the age. Harvest part of the root for medicinal use and replant the rest.

Another Immune System Booster

Barberry

Berberine, the compound that makes goldenseal an immune stimulant and antibiotic, also occurs in barberry (*Berberis vulgaris*), as well as Oregon grape (*Mahonia aquifolium*) and goldthread (*Coptis* species). If you grow barberry as a foundation shrub, you can reap the benefits of goldenseal by making a barberry jelly. Mash 1 cup of barberries, add about ½ cup of water, and simmer until the water evaporates. Add 2 or 3 tablespoons of honey. A more standard way to take barberry is to boil ½ teaspoon of dried root bark in 1 cup of water. *Safety first.* Do not use barberry if you have heart disease or respiratory problems.

HOPS *Humulus lupulus*

Parts used: Female fruits (strobiles)

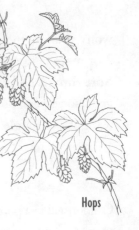

For centuries the ale-loving English looked down on the Germans for using hops to make beer. In about 1500, when English breweries finally did add hops to their traditional sweet ale as a preservative, the bitter taste launched near riots. The herbalist John Gerard later claimed hops were "ill for the head."

Hops

INTERNAL USES

Insomnia. Make an infusion with 2 teaspoons of dried strobiles to 1 cup of water to drink as a nightcap. Or, stuff a pillow with hop strobiles for sweet dreams (see "Make a Hops Pillow" at right).

Sedative. If you're feeling tense and edgy, drink an infusion (2 teaspoons of dried strobiles to 1 cup of water) or take a teaspoon of tincture (1 ounce of herb to 5 ounces of vodka), three times a day.

Indigestion. Hops contain an antispasmodic, so they can quiet a jittery stomach. Use an infusion of 2 teaspoons of dried strobiles to 1 cup of water.

Safety first. Hops are generally very safe, but they can act as a mild depressant, so don't take any if you're already depressed.

Hops Growing Tips

- When the shoots of the hop vine first come up in spring, you can cook and eat them as you would asparagus. They have a nutty taste, but are a bit dry and gritty in texture.
- At the end of the season, remove and compost the dried vine. Heaping plenty of compost on your hop hill before winter will give your vines the rich soil they need and will also blanch the next season's shoots to make them more tender.

When treated right, this perennial vine can grow 25 to 30 feet a year, adding swagger to your herb garden over an entry arch or up a trellis. The lobed leaves, which are up to 5 inches across, look a little like grape leaves. You'll need more than one plant, since they produce male and female flowers separately. The females bear the 1-inch strobiles, which have overlapping papery bracts. Hops need especially rich, loose soil and frequent watering. Plant them in hills, as you would cucumbers or squash. The vine dies to the ground at the end of each season, so no pruning is necessary. *Zones 4–8.*

Make a Hops Pillow

If you have trouble falling asleep, snuggle up with a hops pillow. Simply stitch together two pieces of cotton, leaving an opening on one side large enough to pour in the filling (A). You can make this big enough to replace your regular head pillow, or give it a long, slim shape to fit between two pillows or to slip between your pillow and headboard.

Stuff the pillow full of hops flowers, mixed with a generous amount of lavender and/or rose petals for a sweet scent. Moisten the hops with some glycerine, so they don't rustle and make your insomnia worse instead of better.

If you would like a decorative pillow, make an inner pillow out of plain fabric and a cover out of an attractive print or decorated with lace or appliqué flowers (B).

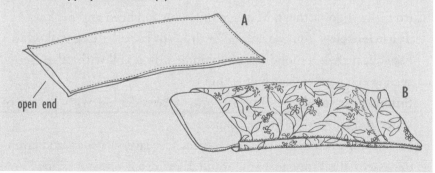

A

open end

B

LAVENDER *Lavandula species*
Parts used: Flowers and leaves

Lavender is a must for any herb gardener, not only for its unique medicinal properties but also for its incredible scent. Aromatherapists say it relaxes and calms at the same time that it lifts depression and fatigue. Lavender essential oil makes a good addition to external herbal remedies that are otherwise rather scentless, such as red pepper salve. (Never take essential oils internally.) There is some evidence that it contains substances that slow pain-transmitting nerve impulses. Don't use Spanish lavender *(L. stoechas)* if you want to relax, though — it tends to be invigorating.

Lavender

INTERNAL USES
Relaxant. You can make a lavender tea to calm your nerves or ease a tension headache. This brew isn't to everyone's taste; in fact, I must admit I think it tastes like perfume. Use 1 teaspoon of the dried leaves and flowers to 1 cup of water.

EXTERNAL USES
Headache. The easiest way to use lavender is to buy the potent essential oil (for external use only), and dilute it by adding a few drops to 1 cup of a base oil, such as almond oil. For headache you can use 5 to 6 drops of lavender essential oil diluted with 1 tablespoon of base oil (to make it go farther). Massage into your forehead and neck.
Tense muscles. You can add a few drops of lavender essential oil to a base oil, such as almond oil, or combine it in an oil with other herbs, such as red pepper, eucalyptus, and mint.
Sunburn or scald. Dilute 20 drops of lavender oil with ½ cup of water and bathe your burned skin.
Insomnia. The possibilities are endless: Use lavender soap, add lavender essential oil to your bath, or put a few drops on your pillow!

There are as many reasons for including lavender in your garden as there are for keeping it in your herbal medicine chest. It makes a pretty underplanting for shrubs such as roses, and can be stunning as the edge to a path. Use the gray foliage and spiky growth habit for dramatic contrast with other plants. Keep a plant in a tall container near a frequently traveled path so that you can sweep your hand through it for a spirit lifter. *Lavandula angustifolia* and *L. latifolia* are the most cold-hardy varieties. All species like slightly alkaline, gritty soil. My friend Nancy McDonald, who gardens in Michigan, plants hers in limestone gravel and snuggles a big rock close to their stems. "I think both the gravel and stone provide extra heat," she says, "so the plants think they're in Greece." Most varieties, *Zones 5–8*.

LEMON BALM *Melissa officinalis*
Parts used: Leaves

"It causeth the mind and heart to become merry," herbalist Nicholas Culpeper wrote in the 17th century, "and driveth away all troublesome cares and thoughts arising from melancholy." Lemon balm may not help you get through an IRS audit, but it is definitely a rewarding plant to grow, exuding the aromas of both mint and lemon. The Greeks noticed that, like many others in the mint family, it's irresistible to bees, and gave it their name for bee, *melissa*.

Lemon Balm

Sedative. Lemon balm contains sedative chemicals called terpenes. Make an infusion of 2 teaspoons of dried lemon balm in 1 cup of hot water before bedtime.

Fevers. A hot infusion promotes sweating that may "break" your fever during a cold. Use 2 teaspoons of the dried herb to 1 cup of water.

Sores and wounds. Lemon balm contains bacteria-fighting compounds. Use an infusion (2 or 3 teaspoons of the dried herb in 1 cup of water) to make a hot compress, or use the leaves as a poultice.

Relaxant. Add lemon balm to your bath by tying a handful of dried leaves in a cloth bag and letting the bathwater run over it.

Cold sores. Studies have found a lemon balm extract useful on cold sores caused by the herpes virus. Make an infusion with 2 or 3 teaspoons of dried leaves per cup of water, and dab it on your cold sores with a cotton ball.

IN THE GARDEN

Unlike others in the mint family, lemon balm does not spread rampantly. Shear it back to keep it from going to seed. Forms that have yellow leaves ('All Gold') and those with variegated leaves ('Variegata') are both useful and ornamental. Give lemon balm a little shade, since it tends to wilt easily, lessening its medicinal properties. *Zones 5–9.*

MEADOWSWEET *Filipendula ulmaria*
Parts used: Leaves and flower tops

You may know that the active ingredient in aspirin, salicin, was originally discovered in the bark of the white willow tree. But the chemists who actually invented aspirin extracted the purer form, salicylic acid, from this beautiful meadow flower. Although meadowsweet contains only small amounts of the pain-relieving chemical, this herb is extremely gentle and won't upset your stomach.

Meadowsweet

INTERNAL USES

Pain relief. Use meadowsweet for headache, muscle pain, menstrual discomfort, and fevers. Because it is so mild, you may get more relief from a tincture than from an infusion. Use 1 part dried herbs to 5 parts vodka or grain alcohol. Take ½ to 1 teaspoon a day.

Ulcers. While aspirin can irritate the stomach lining, studies with animals show that meadowsweet actually protects the stomach from ulcers.

Sometimes called queen-of-the-meadow, this European perennial has such a sweet scent that in the Middle Ages it was scattered on the floors of homes to conceal unpleasant odors. Three to five feet tall with palm-shaped leaves, meadowsweet produces fluffy white plumes in midsummer. A native perennial, *F. rubra*, is even taller, with peachy-pink flowers. Both like damp soil. *Zones 3–9.*

MINT *Mentha × piperita, M. spicata*
Parts used: Leaves and flower tops

Peppermint *(Mentha × piperita)* and spearmint *(M. spicata)* are among the most familiar mints, though you may not think of them as medicines. After-dinner mints are digestive aids and breath fresheners. When you add a commercial inhalant to a vaporizer or rub a drugstore salve on sore muscles, you're getting a dose of menthol, first distilled from peppermint oil about a century ago. Peppermint is generally considered stronger, but you can use spearmint in all the same ways. Not only are mints healing herbs in their own right, but they make useful flavorings for bitter or otherwise unpleasant-tasting herbs.

Peppermint

Spearmint

INTERNAL USE
Digestive aid. To quiet flatulence, quell nausea, and relieve abdominal and gallbladder pains, make an after-dinner mint tea using 2 or 3 teaspoons of dried leaves to 1 cup of water. You can take three or four cups a day. Mint also sweetens the breath.

Safety first. Be careful when giving mint tea to children younger than two. The menthol in it can cause a choking sensation. Try a very dilute tea of about 1 teaspoon of dried leaves to 1 cup water. Pregnant women using mint to alleviate morning sickness should drink only diluted tea and avoid mint altogether if they have any history of miscarriage.

EXTERNAL USE

Decongestant. Add mint leaves to steaming hot water in your bathroom sink, drape a towel over your head, and breathe in the steam to unclog stuffy sinuses. Used in a vaporizer, mint essential oil is excellent for colds, pneumonia, asthma, bronchitis, and laryngitis.

Anesthetic. Because mint has some pain-numbing properties, drug companies often use it in first-aid creams for sunburn and wounds. The leaves make a soothing poultice for either.

Muscle relaxant. Make a massage oil by adding a few drops of the essential oil to a carrier oil such as sweet almond.

IN THE GARDEN

Mint has a reputation as a real thug in the garden, spreading ruthlessly and muscling out milder-mannered plants. Since it's merely pleasant to look at but not a dazzler, keep it in solitary confinement. You can

Minty-Fresh Ideas

- **Insect repellent.** Mint is a pleasant-smelling and surprisingly effective insect repellent. Make a mint sachet and hang it on a porch to control flies or in a closet to discourage moths. Put a few drops of mint essential oil where you suspect ants are gaining entry to your home.
- **Waker-upper.** American colonists used mint to get the bugs out of their thought processes, too. Because the fresh, bright scent clears the head and rejuvenates the spirit, they kept jars of mint potpourri on their work desks.

attempt to hem it in with metal, plastic, brick, or boards sunk at least 6 inches into the ground. I find it easier to keep mine in a large pot, which I move to cover temporary bare spots in my flower bed. Repot it, or divide and move it every four or five years, since it gets woody in the center and depletes the nutrients in the soil. Keep the tops trimmed off to make it bushier, but once flowers do start to form, harvest all the above-ground parts, leaving the stems just a few inches tall. *Zones 5–9.*

MULLEIN *Verbascum thapsus*
Parts used: Leaves, flowers, and roots

European settlers picked up a lot of herbal tips from Native Americans, but with mullein the tables were probably turned. The Europeans brought this towering biennial with them, and made dye with the roots and candlewicks with the stems (or dipped the whole flower spike in suet and turned it into a torch), and stuffed the leaves in their socks to keep their feet warm. They also prized mullein for respiratory problems: They cooked the root with molasses for sore throats and smoked the dried leaves for coughs and colds.

Mullein

INTERNAL USES
Respiratory problems. Mullein contains mucilage, which swells when it gets wet and forms a soothing gel. It's also an expectorant, helping to expel mucus from the upper respiratory tract. Herbalists recommend it for bronchitis, sore throat, cold and flu, coughs, laryngitis, and allergies. Use 1 or 2 teaspoons of mullein per cup of water. The flowers are especially powerful. If you use roots as well, boil them for about 10 minutes and then turn off the heat, add the flowers and leaves, and allow them to steep, then strain. The tea is bitter, so you'll want to add your favorite flavoring to make it palatable.
Safety first. Do not use the seeds, which are toxic.

Hemorrhoids. Mullein is both an astringent and an emollient; it contracts the skin as well as soothes it. Use 1 teaspoon of dried herbs steeped in ½ cup of vinegar combined with ½ cup of water. Apply it to hemorrhoids with a compress.

Earache. Make a cold infusion of crushed mullein flowers and olive oil. Use eardrops only when your doctor has assured you the eardrum is not perforated.

Irritated skin. Make a cold infusion or salve to treat itchy skin or minor burns.

IN THE GARDEN

"O for a lute of fire to sing their praises," Henry Mitchell, the *Washington Post*'s late garden columnist, wrote of the *Verbascum* clan. Only moderately amazing the first year, when they form rosettes of felty foliage (*Verbascum* is sometimes called flannel plant), they become rockets the next year, shooting up 3- to 6-foot gray spikes into which yellow flowers seem to be tucked at random. *V. thapsus,* the species-with-a-thousand-uses, easily becomes invasive, so other

Marsh Mallow Treats

Plants like mullein that contain mucilage get gooey when soaked. Another familiar plant with this characteristic is marsh mallow (*Althaea officinalis*). You can pulverize its roots and mix them with water to smear on cuts and scrapes for a soothing effect. You can also use 1 teaspoon of the dried root to make a decoction to drink for a sore throat. Grocery store marshmallows no longer contain this herb, but you can make the original treat by peeling some root, boiling it until soft, and soaking it in a thick syrup made of equal parts of sugar and water. Cool the pieces on a waxed-paper-lined cookie sheet.

Marsh mallow

varieties (such as *V. bombyciferum, V. olympicum,* and *V. chaixii)* are more often invited into gardens. If you're diligent, you can prevent much of the self-sowing by harvesting the flowers before they set seed.

PARSLEY *Petroselinum crispum*
Parts used: Leaves, seeds, and roots

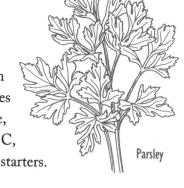
Parsley

Parsley, ho-hum. It's the garnish that most Americans spurn when it appears on their plates in restaurants. But when it comes to nutrition, parsley makes spinach pale, replete as it is with protein, vitamins A and C, calcium, magnesium, and potassium, just for starters.

INTERNAL USES

Urinary tract problems. Diuretic herbs keep our body's plumbing running smoothly by causing it to produce more urine, and prevent problems such as kidney stones and bladder infections. They also relieve bloating during menstruation. Make an infusion with 2 or more teaspoons of dried leaves, or a decoction with 2 teaspoons of root or 1 teaspoon of seeds per cup of water.

Bad breath. There's a reason for that parsley on the edge of your dinner plate: It's an effective breath freshener. Munch on it.

Safety first. Parsley contains a chemical called apiol, which is sold in Russia to start labor. Don't use it medicinally if you are pregnant.

IN THE GARDEN

Every gardener should grow parsley to feed the larvae of beautiful swallowtail butterflies. This biennial grows a foot tall and can have flat (that's the more flavorful Italian parsley) or curly leaves. The small yellow flowers grow in airy, flat-topped clusters. Cookbooks advise you to harvest all your parsley the first year, since the flavor goes downhill once it flowers. But for herbal medicine, you'll want to keep it around to harvest seeds the second year.

RED PEPPER *Capsicum annuum, C. frutescens*

Parts used: Fruit

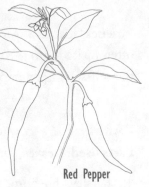

Red Pepper

It may come as a surprise that a plant so hot can be used as a massage ointment to relieve pain. Scientists say that the capsaicin in peppers gradually depletes a pain transmitter called substance P. By mildly irritating the skin, capsaicin increases blood flow and speeds healing. The more potent the pepper, the greater its medicinal value. Taken internally, it stimulates the natural painkillers called endorphins.

INTERNAL USES

Digestive aid. Instead of giving you heartburn, red pepper actually stimulates the flow of saliva and stomach secretions.

Weight loss. According to one British study, 2 teaspoons of red pepper sauce a day cranks up your metabolism 25 percent and helps burn calories. If you don't have a tolerance for hot spice, add ½ teaspoon to a glass of tomato juice and drink 4 glasses a day.

Other uses. Research shows that peppers may lower cholesterol and the risk of blood clots. A diet rich in peppers may also help ease chronic arthritic or rheumatic pain, and combat fatigue.

Safety first. When chopping hot peppers, wear gloves, slip plastic bags over your hands, or use vinegar or lemon juice to wash the capsaicin off your hands. To avoid burning your eyes, don't touch your face or eyes with this substance on your hands. If that happens, flush them repeatedly with cold water.

EXTERNAL USES

Muscle pain, backache, and arthritis. Treat yourself to a massage using a salve or an ointment made with a decoction of red peppers. Start with ½ teaspoon of dried crushed peppers in 1 cup of vegetable oil, such as safflower or grapeseed oil. Adjust the amount up or down according to your preference. Add a few drops of your favorite essential oil to create a more fragrant experience.

Cluster headaches. A recent study found a red pepper ointment effective for these chronic headaches, which are rarer than migraines and occur primarily in men. As a preventive measure, purchase capsicum capsules and follow the directions on the package.

IN THE GARDEN

Easy and beautiful to grow, many hot peppers are worthy of inclusion in ornamental gardens. Long and slim or small and round, peppers range in color from bright red and near yellow, to orange and even purple. Southern gardeners can sow them directly in the ground, but in other climates you need to start them indoors in winter. Red peppers don't require rich soil, although they do need full sun.

ROSEMARY *Rosmarinus officinalis*
Parts used: Leaves

In the language of flowers, rosemary means remembrance. Because rosemary helps food stay fresh — it contains a powerful preservative — the ancients decided it might also keep things fresh in our minds. Modern research shows that rosemary contains antioxidants, which defend us against the free radicals that cause aging. So, rosemary may help preserve us, too!

Rosemary

Memory enhancement and anti-aging. Traditional use and recent studies show rosemary may prevent memory loss and may retard other aging processes as well. Make an infusion with 1 teaspoon of leaves to 1 cup of water and drink up to three times a day.

Other uses. Traditional uses also include aiding digestion and breaking up congestion. Use as described above.

Useful Weeds

When you weed your garden, of course you compost any weeds that don't have seeds. But take a second look at the following common backyard weeds. Here's a triplet that you may wish to add to your herbal medicine chest:

- Dandelion *(Taraxacum officinale)* is a liver tonic. Make a decoction using 1 teaspoon of dried root to 1 cup of water. Drink up to 3 cups a day.

- Plantain *(Plantago major)* leaves can take the sting out of poison ivy, insect bites, and other skin injuries. Apply fresh leaves as a poultice. Both the leaves and seeds of this common weed contain mucilage that makes a gentle laxative. Psyllium, which is used in commercial preparations such as Metamucil, is a related plant.

- Purslane *(Portulaca oleracea)* contains omega-3 fatty acids and antioxidants that prevent heart disease. Make this part of your diet, raw in salads or steamed.

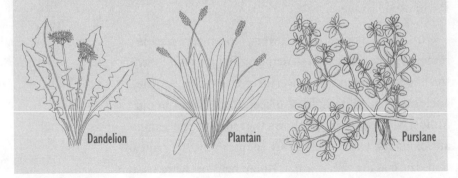

Dandelion   Plantain   Purslane

Infection prevention. Rosemary has antibacterial properties. Add it to salves for wounds, or use fresh leaves as a poultice on minor cuts.

Mouthwash and gargle. Rosemary and myrrh are an especially effective combination for treating a sore throat. Rosemary also helps stop bad breath. Infuse 2 teaspoons of dried rosemary in 1 cup of water.

Aromatherapy. Rosemary lifts depression and relieves anxiety, so it's a good herb for the bath, massage oils, and cosmetics. And its antibacterial properties help eliminate body odor.

IN THE GARDEN

It's easy to see why all kinds of pleasant things, such as love charms and sweet dreams, were attributed to this distinctively fragrant little shrub with its bright blue flowers. Rosemary requires more warmth and drainage than most Mediterranean culinary herbs. North of Zone 8, you will need to bring it indoors for the winter, although 'Arp' is a cold-tolerant cultivar that can survive most Zone 7 winters. Keep rosemary on a windowsill facing south, taking care not to overwater it. Mist it once in awhile, but let it go completely dry between waterings. Rosemary can reach a height exceeding 3 feet. *Zones 8–10.*

SAGE *Salvia officinalis*
Parts used: Leaves

Sage is another common herb garden plant. It's so potent you'll have a hard time using great quantities of it for cooking, so consider employing some leaves to treat gardening injuries or incorporating them in antiperspirants. Sage is a good food preservative and source of antioxidants, but it is not safe for long-term medicinal use.

Sage

INTERNAL USE

Memory aid and anti-aging. Use 1 teaspoon of the dried herb per cup of water, and take up to 2 cups per day.

Other uses. Studies in Japan have isolated a compound in an Asian sage, *S. militiorrhiza*, that could be an effective, nonaddictive tranquilizer. Sage tea may also minimize night sweats and hot flashes.

Safety first. Sage contains thujone, which can cause convulsions if taken in large amounts. Sage is not safe for regular long-term medicinal use.

EXTERNAL USES

Sore throat. The tannins in sage are good for the throat and gums. Steep 2 teaspoons of finely chopped sage in 1 cup of water for a mouthwash or gargle, or drink it for a sore throat.

Gingivitis. Brushing your teeth and gums with a rough-textured sage leaf is refreshing and stimulating, plus it freshens your breath. The tannins and antiseptic compounds help heal bleeding gums.

Canker sores. Sage's antibacterial properties make it an effective treatment for canker sores. Make a tea with 2 teaspoons of dried herb to 1 cup of water and rinse your mouth with it.

Antiperspirant. To halve perspiration, make a tincture with ½ teaspoon dried sage in 1 cup vodka. Use cotton balls to apply it to your underarms two or three times a day. It starts working in about 2 hours.

Other uses. A sage infusion may help get rid of dandruff.

Controlling Coughs

If coughing accompanies your sore throat, you'll be glad to know about horehound as well as sage. The leaves and flowers of this perennial mint have helped ease coughs for at least 400 years, and horehound candy was a stock item in drugstores of yesteryear. The round, wrinkled leaves are woolly, setting off more colorful plants, but you'll want to set firm boundaries for it, like the rest of the mint clan. Try an infusion of 2 teaspoons of dried leaves in a cup of water with honey and lemon.

Horehound

When the striking blue flowers are spent, the leathery leaves still make sage an ornamental standout. After it flowers, trim off any branches that have become ragged and bare to stimulate new growth. Sage is easy to start from seeds or by layering. Just pin the center of a branch into the soil with a hairpin-style wire, and the stem will take root in two or three weeks. Then you can cut it from the mother plant and replant elsewhere — or give it to a friend. Sage can turn into a small shrub, more than 3 feet tall and 2 feet wide. Provide it with full sun and good drainage, and divide it every four years. *Zones 4–9.*

St.-John's-Wort *Hypericum perforatum*
Parts used: Flowers and leaves

St.-John's-wort is one of the best-known herbal medicines in the United States. While it's typically used to lift mild depression, *Hypericum's* active ingredients can also heal bruises and burns, and boost the immune system; it's also being investigated as treatment for the HIV virus and AIDS.

St.-John's-Wort

INTERNAL USE
Depression. If you tend to get mild cases of the blues, St.-John's-wort might help. To make your own preparation, steep 1 or 2 teaspoons of the dried herb in 1 cup of boiling water for 10 minutes. You can take one or two cups a day for four to six weeks. If you purchase capsules, follow instructions on the package of a standardized extract. *Safety first. Don't treat your own depression if you have severe or long-lasting mood swings, or if you take other medication for depression. Internal use can make fair-skinned people extremely sensitive to the sun.*

EXTERNAL USES
Bruises and sores. Make a tincture or buy one containing standardized extract. Apply the tincture directly to your injury or dilute it with

water and use with a compress. You can also apply the fresh, crushed leaves and flowers as a poultice.

IN THE GARDEN

St.-John's-wort got its common name because the flowers bloom around St. John's Day, June 24, and the red oil from its flowers and red spots on its leaves were said to be the blood of the martyr.

There are several handsome species and cultivars of this woody perennial, ranging from ground covers to good-sized shrubs. Especially popular with Northwest gardeners, most have yellow flowers with prominent stamens. *H. perforatum* (the focus of nearly all the research on the plant's use as an antidepressant) is an extremely aggressive spreader that smells like paint remover. Like most invasive plants, St.-John's-wort grows in almost any soil, in both sun and shade.

If you are making your own herbal preparation of St.-John's-wort, use fresh flowers and leaves if possible; this herb loses its effectiveness more rapidly than other herbs when dried and stored. Its shelf life is not more than 6 months. *Zones 3–8.*

THYME *Thymus vulgaris*
Parts used: Leaves

If you have ever had the good fortune to walk through a field of wild thyme, it is a sensory experience you will never forget. The Romans praised it as an antidote to melancholy. Charlemagne ordered it grown in his imperial gardens. As a symbol of courage, medieval noblewomen embroidered sprigs of thyme on the silken scarves their knights carried off to the Crusades. Shakespeare rhapsodized over its fragrant joys. A favorite of the bees, a delight to the gardener and cook, and a necessity to the herbalist, thyme has been a culinary and medicinal staple since time immemorial.

Thyme

Digestive aid. Steep 2 teaspoons of the dried herb in 1 cup of hot water to relieve gassiness and ease a queasy stomach.

Cough suppressant. Thyme relaxes the muscles of the windpipe and loosens phlegm, so this herb eases symptoms of bronchitis. Make an infusion, as described above, and sweeten with honey.

Pain relief. Thyme contains thymol, which increases blood flow to the skin. The warmth is comforting, and some herbalists feel that the increased blood flow speeds healing. You'll find it in a lot of commercial products. Add a thyme infusion to your homemade salves.

Antiseptic. Used as a poultice, thyme's bacterial- and fungus-fighting properties aid healing.

Antidepressant. Aromatherapists say thyme's scent is a mood lifter.

Over 300 thyme species include some with yellow or multicolored leaves, creeping and shrub-type thymes, lemon-scented or sage-scented ones, thymes with woolly leaves and leaves the size of pinheads, and plants with white, pink, or purple flowers. Let it cascade from a strawberry jar or poke into rock gardens. *Zones 5–8.*

VALERIAN *Valeriana officinalis*

Parts used: Rhizome and root, powdered

You probably learned that the Pied Piper lured away the children of Hamelin with his sparkling personality and musical prowess. But the oldest versions of the story attribute his charms to hypnotic valerian. It was once used for treating epilepsy, and then was brought into service against shell shock during World War I. Much like catnip, valerian excites felines but calms human beings. Of all the herbs we can take to unwind, valerian is the most powerful.

Valerian

Mild tranquilizer and sleep aid. Make a decoction with 2 teaspoons of the powdered root to 1 cup of water. Valerian's unpleasant smell and taste led ancient Greeks to call it *phu.* Add lemon or other herbs to make it more palatable.

Safety first. Do not take valerian with any other sedatives. Never use with alcohol.

IN THE GARDEN

Valerian is sometimes called garden heliotrope, and like that annual it is strongly scented. Most people compare the aroma to vanilla. A 5-foot-tall perennial, it has somewhat fernlike leaves, and the flat-topped flowers are usually white, although they can also be pink or lavender. You can harvest the big taproots in the fall of its second year for medicinal purposes, dividing off some to replant. (The "phu" smell develops as the roots dry.) If you're lucky, it will also self-sow — but you may have to fence it to keep cats from loving it to death. *Zones 4–8.*

WILLOW *Salix species*

Parts used: Bark and, less powerfully, leaves

The Chinese used willow bark to relieve pain some 2,500 years ago. Native Americans were fighting fever with willow-root steam baths and willow tea when the Pilgrims landed. In the 1820s, Western scientists extracted the active ingredient, salicin, from the white willow, *S. alba.* Willow bark is much gentler on the system than

Willow

aspirin is. Purdue University professor emeritus Varro Tyler estimates that you may need up to 20 teaspoons a day to get the same benefits, but he feels that willow contains too much tannin to be safe in those amounts. Other herbalists disagree that such a large dose is required. If you experience no side effects from aspirin, try willow for pain and fever and see if it works for you.

Tea (Camellia sinensis)

When most of us talk about tea, we're thinking of an iced or hot drink made from the leaves of *Camellia sinensis*. Commonly called tea plant, it is a less showy relative of the evergreen shrubs whose blossoms light up southern gardens in winter. The beverage made from its leaves is more than just an alternative to coffee: Like willow, it can help prevent stroke, and it also helps lower cholesterol, enhances liver function, and can be used to treat congestion, diarrhea, and tooth decay. All green, oolong, and black teas are made from this Asian shrub.

Tea

INTERNAL USES

Pain and fever. Make a decoction by simmering 1 teaspoon of powdered bark in 1 cup of water for about ½ hour. Drink this for headache, backache, muscle aches, the pain from arthritis, or the discomfort and fever of colds and flu. Add an emollient such as marsh mallow or plantain to help prevent possible stomach irritation.

Preventing heart attack and stroke. Some physicians recommend low daily doses of aspirin to prevent blood clots, which can have life-threatening consequences. You might try mixing a teaspoon of willow bark in a more pleasant-tasting herbal tea. But talk to your doctor before you decide to take willow bark every day.

Safety first. Don't use willow bark if aspirin has ever given you any problems. In addition to an upset stomach, it can cause tinnitus (ringing in the ears).

IN THE GARDEN

The big white willow is always mentioned as the source of salicin, but there are other showy species that contain even more of the active ingredient. *Salix daphnoides* is called the violet willow for its purple new bark; *S. fragilis* has reddish wood and is called crack willow because its branches snap off easily; and *S. purpurea,* or purple osier, has extremely narrow twigs used for basket making. All of these species have cultivars with weeping habits or golden winter twigs. To harvest the bark, trim off a mature branch and strip its bark, or, in the fall, remove bark carefully from only one side of the tree (never strip bark all the way around a tree or you will kill it).

WITCH HAZEL
Hamamelis virginiana
Parts used: Leaves, bark, and twigs

Witch Hazel

Here's an herb that you probably know, but more for the end product than the plant. Colonists used the supple branches of this native American shrub as divining rods to search for water and to make broom handles. Many people believe that because we associate witches with brooms, witch hazel is named for these sorceresses.

According to Michael Castleman, author of *The Healing Herbs,* however, the flexibility of the branches explains the common name: In Middle English the word *wich* means "flexible." Native Americans treated muscle aches and black eyes with witch hazel decoctions and steam baths. To buy a full-strength tincture, purchase witch hazel at a health food store. The commercial witch hazel sold in pharmacies today is made through steam distillation, which removes the tannins, but it is still valuable as an antiseptic and astringent.

EXTERNAL USES
Body aches and pains. Make an infusion with 1 teaspoon of leaves or a decoction with 1 teaspoon of ground twigs per cup of water. Use it to give a massage, or apply as a compress.

Bruises and bites. Make a poultice of leaves and powdered bark. You may find that it also reduces swelling.

Hemorrhoids. Witch hazel is an active ingredient in many commercial salves. A compress of a commercial extract or homemade witch hazel concoction can ease pain and itching. Commercial witch hazel contains some rubbing alcohol. If your hemorrhoids are bleeding, you may find that the witch hazel will cause a bit of stinging.

Tired eyes. I always knew when my grandmother had a hard day, because she would rest for a few minutes in a dark bedroom, eyes closed and covered with cotton pads saturated (but not dripping) with witch hazel. The smell makes me nostalgic, and it's relaxing as well.

IN THE GARDEN

This low-growing tree, with several related species and cultivars, can be a wonderful addition to your garden. The spidery, lightly fragrant flowers will cheer you in late fall and even into midwinter.

The native species, *H. virginiana*, at 20 feet tall, is probably the biggest, with an equally wide spread. It has yellow fall flowers.

Hybrids and cultivars have pale yellow, orange, and red flowers that bloom in January and February, making these one of the earliest welcome signs of spring in many regions. *Zones 4–8.*

A Witch for Your Itch

Steven Foster, author of *Herbal Renaissance*, treats poison ivy with a homemade witch hazel tincture that he makes this way: In winter, gather five or six 3-foot-long branches and scrape off the bark. Use a kitchen scale to weigh the bark, then add twice that amount in vodka. Let it set two weeks, shaking it daily. Strain the tincture into a dark bottle. Store up to 1 year in a cool, dark place.

YARROW *Achillea millefolium*

Parts used: Flower tops, leaves, and stems

Achilles (the Greek hero with the fragile heel) used a relative of this familiar fernlike plant to stop the bleeding of his wounded soldiers. Yarrow has never lost its reputation; in fact, one of its common names is woundwort. Yarrow is full of active compounds that work three ways on wounds — they help blood to clot, relieve pain and swelling, and kill germs.

Yarrow

INTERNAL USES

Digestive aid. Infusions of yarrow flowers stimulate gastric juices. Drink up to three cups a day.

Sedative. Infusions of the flowers may also work as a mild sedative and to relieve menstrual cramps. Drink up to three cups a day.

Safety first. Drinking yarrow can turn urine brown, but this is a normal reaction, not cause for worry.

EXTERNAL USES

Cuts, scrapes, and bruises. Use fresh yarrow leaves and flowers as a poultice, or make an infusion or tincture to use as a compress. Use 1 or 2 teaspoons of dried herbs per cup of water for an infusion, or 1 ounce of dried yarrow and 5 ounces of alcohol for a tincture.

IN THE GARDEN

Achillea millefolium, a European perennial in the aster family, has joined other exuberant nonnatives such as bachelor buttons and Queen Anne's lace on U.S. roadsides. Plants that naturalize readily usually need little care, and yarrow is no exception. It likes moderately fertile soil and full sun, and benefits from being divided now and then. Three feet tall, it has feathery foliage and off-white flower clusters that are well worth picking for fresh or dried arrangements. *Zones 3–9.*

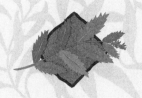

CHAPTER 4

GROWING
Healing Herbs

Most medicinal herbs are incredibly easy to grow and have a long history of use as garden plants. When you nurture plentiful mounds of lavender and lemon balm, with perhaps a big clump of meadowsweet toward the back of a shady bed and some thyme between stepping-stones, you're sharing the pleasure of gardeners several centuries back, who also loved the exuberant fragrance of these herbs. If you decide to attract bees and butterflies to your yard, you'll find that coneflower and hyssop are a must. When company comes, take them on a stroll through your garden and share stories about your plants. Nothing beats herbs for horticultural lore — both fact and legend.

While herbs are beautiful additions to many gardens, most modern gardeners have lost touch with herbs' healing traditions and potential. Growing your own medicinal herbs brings an added dimension of satisfaction to gardening, because you know that your healthy soil, as well as the great exercise you get tending your garden, means better health for you and your family. Some medicinal herbs are well-suited for small gardens; others enhance shady gardens and some even prefer boggy conditions. A medicinal herb garden can be as exquisitely formal as an Elizabethan knot garden or as joyously informal as an English cottage garden. You can also weave medicinal herbs among your vegetables, choosing them as companion plants to help ward off garden pests. You might want to use them in a perennial border as accents or snuggled at the feet of showier garden plants. Whatever style you choose, as with any plants, the key to success lies in matching your growing conditions to each herb's needs.

Here are some tips to consider and some advice about how to create your own medicinal herb garden.

Creating a Home for Your New Garden

You will be able to grow the widest array of herbs if you give them excellent drainage and full sun — which means at least 6 hours of sun a day. Under these conditions, most herbs produce the most concentrated volatile oils and, importantly, their most potent healing compounds. Between drainage and sun, drainage is the more important. Although a few herbs, such as marsh mallow, prefer boggy conditions, most need oxygen around their roots in order to remain healthy. Don't despair if your garden is somewhat shady. Many herbs do just as well in part shade, and others "tolerate shade," which means they will survive, even though they may not be as large or bloom as flamboyantly. One advantage to light shade, especially in the South, is that the plants require less watering during a summer drought.

Microclimates. In deciding the best site for your new garden of healing herbs, keep in mind that every spot has its own microclimate. Even a small garden has areas that are wetter or drier, hotter or cooler, sunnier or shadier than their surroundings. A northern exposure, especially on a hill, will frost later in spring and earlier in fall than the rest of the garden. In an eastern exposure, herbs are treated to gentler morning sun with shady afternoons. Fortunately, some like it hot, and Mediterranean herbs can tolerate a southern or western exposure's harsher afternoon sun. A brick wall or white fence reflects additional warmth and will protect your herbs from the wind. And speaking of wind, observe the direction from which it blows most frequently and avoid exposing marginally hardy or very tall plants to its onslaught. Remember, too, that plants may get cold, wet feet at the bottom of a slope, where both frigid air and rainwater settle. On the other hand, herbs planted under the eaves of your house will receive almost no rain.

Width of beds. Think about how you will get your hands on your plants to tend and harvest them. Most people find it uncomfortable to lean out even a couple of feet for any period of time (as you would when weeding), so a 3-foot-wide bed that you can reach from both sides is ideal. If your bed is wider, place some stepping-stones among the plants so you can reach your herbs without trampling on your nice fluffy garden soil. You don't have to buy slate or flagstone pavers. Salvaged flat chunks of concrete are great for this purpose.

Garden paths. Whenever you are adding new beds to a landscape, you should plan your paths before you put seeds or plants in the ground. They should be wide enough so that you can hunker down on them with your herb harvesting tools. Every type of paving material has pros and cons. Brick is traditional, and stepping-stones and pavers are handsome, but both require some skill and labor to lay properly. Gravel is less expensive, but often gets kicked into the planting beds. I like shredded wood mulch because I get it free from my county, it's cool and soft to walk on, and it breaks down to improve the soil. Its one disadvantage is that I have to replace it each year.

TAKING TIME TO PREPARE THE SITE

You'll be more satisfied with your herb garden in the long run if you take the time to plan and prepare it right. If your site is covered with heavy sod, you may decide to rent a sod stripper — which is about the size of a lawnmower — to remove it. If the area is mostly weeds, it's best to get rid of them as completely as you can before you put in a garden. The box below contains some suggestions for approaches you can take to remove turf and weeds.

Zapping Your Weeds

In summer, you can kill weeds in a sunny spot by using a technique called solarization. Till and water the site, then cover the area with 6 to 8 mil, clear plastic. Hold down the plastic with stones, brick, lumber, or even mounds of soil. The weeds should bake to death in about a month.

You can also smother weeds with black plastic, cardboard, or layers of newspapers held down with straw. Cardboard and newspaper will eventually decompose and add their fiber to your soil, but this method can take several months or all winter long. Often you'll be so eager to begin your new garden that you won't want to put up with this waiting period. If you remove the plastic or paper after just a few weeks, a new generation of weed seedlings may erupt, but you should be able to hack out these shallow-rooted weeds with a brisk hoeing or hand-held cultivator.

Solarizing soil

TESTING THE SOIL FOR SUCCESS

If the site you choose has not had a recent soil test, do one now to be sure that the soil has the nutrients your plants will need and that its pH (acidity or alkalinity) is the proper level. Most herbs require a neutral range — 6.5 to 7.2. Purchase a soil-testing kit or send a sample to a government or private testing agency. Ask your local garden center or county extension service for advice about services near you; they are usually listed under county government in your phone book. Be sure to tell them you want to use organic amendments. You'll receive a report that advises you about what to add to correct any nutrient deficiencies. Depending on the results, you can use fish emulsion to increase the nitrogen content in your soil, wood ash for potassium, and bone meal for phosphorus.

Even if you don't test your soil, you'll want to add 2 or 3 inches of organic matter, such as compost, aged manure, or leaf mold, to improve the texture and structure of your soil. If you have heavy clay, amending it generously with organic matter will increase the space between soil particles.

Adding sand to your clay will not solve the problem, and may only make it more cementlike. If you have sandy soil to begin with, organic amendments will help bind the soil particles together, hold moisture, and provide plants with additional nutrients.

Coping with Weeds from Compost

Remember that unless you keep your compost hot and steaming until its contents are "cooked," any seeds in it can still sprout and you may be spreading weeds on your garden site along with the compost. Weed sprouts don't have to be a problem if you can put off planting for two weeks or so. As you wait, if any seeds germinate, simply hoe them down.

DESIGNS THAT WORK

Deciding how to arrange your plants in the bed is one of the most creative, personal, and satisfying aspects of gardening. You can match flower and foliage colors, or choose contrasting options. Tall plants can go in the back of the bed, fronted by shorter ones, or you can place them off to one side as an accent. Plants like fennel and angelica have tall, dramatic foliage and can be used as accents or centerpieces.

The best part of garden design is that nothing's permanent, so you don't have to worry about making mistakes. If your first effort doesn't leave you breathless, you can easily move perennial herbs around in the fall and spring, and annuals are a whole new show every year.

A BACKYARD HERB GARDEN

Even a medium-sized yard can provide you with enough microclimates to play host to herbs that require a wide range of conditions. The garden at the right is based on my own backyard herb garden, but you may find you have some of these features in your yard, too. A slope on the northern side of my patio makes a good place for wetland herbs such as willow and meadowsweet. Regardless of the layout of your yard, try a long-raised bed, as I have done for rosemary, lavender, catnip, and other herbs that need excellent drainage. The raised bed also makes it easy to harvest herbs for both healing and cooking.

Consider grouping herbs with an eye toward the ornamental, too. I've grouped medicinal herbs with yellow and purple flowers, many of which have gray-green foliage, on the sunny eastern side of my yard, and together they make a lovely — and fragrant — display. If you have room, consider a trellis for hops and a few taller medicinal herbs such as witch hazel or chaste tree to create a privacy screen.

A NATIVE AMERICAN HEALING HERBS GARDEN

Even if you can't grow all the medicinal herbs you'd like, an area devoted to herbs will help you feel more in touch with their powerful healing traditions. The garden on page 82, which features herbs used by Native Americans, tolerates a lot of shade and makes a mini-retreat.

Backyard Herb Garden

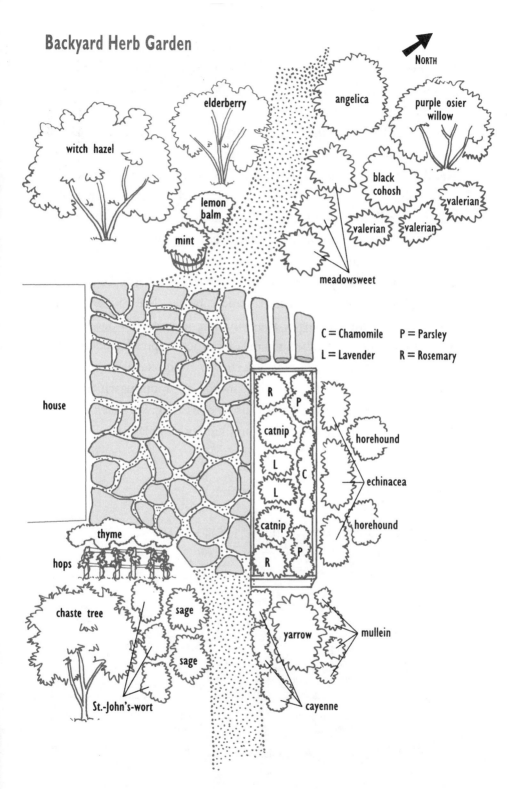

NORTH

witch hazel

elderberry

angelica

purple osier willow

lemon balm

black cohosh

valerian

mint

valerian valerian

meadowsweet

C = Chamomile   P = Parsley

L = Lavender   R = Rosemary

house

R   P

catnip

horehound

L   C

L

echinacea

catnip

horehound

R   P

thyme

hops

chaste tree

sage

sage

yarrow

mullein

St.-John's-wort

cayenne

Many of the herbs in this design are discussed in Chapter 3, "Essential Healing Herbs A to Z," which begins on page 27. We've added a few others that were traditionally used by Native Americans and that are easy to find and grow.

Bayberry *(Myrica cerifera)*. Choctaws used leaves and stems of this aromatic broad-leaved evergreen shrub for fever.

Bearberry *(Arctostaphylos uva-ursi)*. The women of several tribes used this trailing shrub (which grows mainly in the northeastern United States) to relieve discomfort during menstruation and labor, as well as for urinary system problems. Today, studies focus on its use against herpes, flu, and dental plaque.

Passionflower *(Passiflora incarnata)*. Native Americans used a poultice of passionflower root for boils, cuts, and earaches. Tea from any part of the plant is a mild sedative. Passionflower is beautiful, but this vine grows to 30 feet and can become invasive when it spreads underground.

Wintergreen *(Gaultheria procumbens)*. Wintergreen is a member of the heath family. It is low growing and bears drooping white flowers and red berries. Native Americans use wintergreen tea for colds, headaches, stomach aches, fevers, and kidney complaints.

Native American Medicinal Herb Garden

HEALING HERBS IN CONTAINERS

Almost any plant except huge trees can be grown for at least several seasons in a container. The biggest difference between container gardening and gardening in the ground is that your container plants usually require more frequent watering than plants in a garden bed. Most of the plants in the groupings suggested here, with the possible exception of mint, can tolerate quite a bit of dryness. It's essential that they have excellent drainage, since it's easy for water to accumulate in the bottom of containers and kill plants by rotting their roots.

Try grouping herbs by symptom in a large container, such as a half-whiskey barrel, good-sized window box, or a strawberry jar. Here are a few possibilities:

Cold and Flu Herbs

Headache. Red pepper, feverfew, lavender, lemon balm

Cold, flu, sore throat, and other respiratory problems. Garlic, horehound, sage, thyme

Digestive problems. Chamomile, lemon balm, mint, rosemary, yarrow

Sedative herbs. Chamomile, lemon balm, lavender, catnip

Digestive Herbs

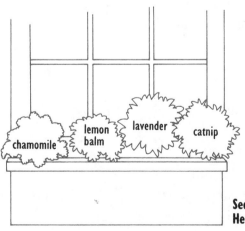

Sedative Herbs

STARTING HERB PLANTS FROM SEED

Getting a piece of matter that looks as lifeless as a grain of sand to swell, root, and develop into a complex, self-sustaining organism is a truly awe-inspiring phenomenon. What's just as intriguing is that it's so easy to get the process going. You can sow seeds indoors to get a head start on the season, or wait and plant them directly in the ground where they will grow. Outdoors, plan your sowing so that the seeds won't sprout until after the average last frost date in your region. Be sure to keep your seedbed moist from the time you sow until the seedlings are several inches tall. Indoors, in order to keep seedlings growing and healthy until you can safely move them outside, the most important requirements are a clean environment and as much light as possible.

Seed-starting containers. For indoor seed starting, you have your choice of many different containers, both recycled and purchased for the purpose. A good choice is a seed-starter kit that includes a bottom tray, individual seed cells, and a clear plastic dome. These can be sterilized and reused for two or three seasons, and the dome creates a humid environment that speeds germination.

If you use recycled containers, achieve the same greenhouse effect by covering them with plastic bags or plastic wrap. Puncture the bottom of recycled containers so that excess water can drain away, and place containers

Herbs to Grow from Seed

Calendula

Catnip

Chaste tree

Evening primrose

Fennel

Feverfew

German chamomile

Horehound

Hyssop

Lemon balm

Mullein

Parsley

Red pepper

Sage

Valerian

Yarrow

Providing drainage holes

- Before you sow, sterilize your seed-starting trays in a solution that contains 1 part household bleach to 9 parts water. Rinse them in clear water before filling them with seed-starting mix.
- Avoid damping-off, the biggest enemy of young seedlings, by using a sterile seed-starting mix, not garden soil, which can be full of disease organisms. (Damping-off is a fungal disease that rots seedlings at the base.)
- Before sowing the seeds, wet the planting medium thoroughly with hot water, until it is evenly moist but not soaking wet.

in a shallow pan or tray. After the seedlings germinate, remove the plastic covering to allow good air circulation.

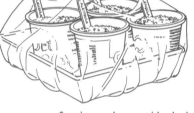

Covering seed trays with plastic

Planting depth. Although a seed-starting rule of thumb is to plant seeds to twice their depth, this doesn't mean you have to bring out a ruler. Most seeds are bound and determined to find their way to the surface. If you are working with extremely tiny seeds, or seeds described as needing light to germinate, just sprinkle them on the surface of the soil, then pat them down gently, as if you were saying goodnight to a baby.

Watering. Water just enough to keep soil moist. To avoid disease problems, and to keep from capsizing small seedlings, water by filling the bottom tray with enough water to soak up through the drainage holes. You can also use a plant mister to keep the planting medium wet enough for germination.

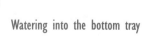

Watering into the bottom tray

Labels. Remember to label all trays and rows! You may think you'll remember where you planted each herb and recognize it as it develops, but that's not always the case. Small wooden or plastic stakes make the best labels. Test your marking pen to make sure that it's waterproof; a waterproof fine-point pen, for example, is excellent.

Light. A sunny windowsill will give seeds sufficient light until they germinate. Once they do, seedlings need 12 to 16 hours of light a day, and reaching for light from a windowsill makes them leggy. Place your seed trays under grow lights, which provide sunlike, full-spectrum light of the proper intensity for good seedling growth. The tops of the plants should be no farther than 4 inches from the light source.

Transplanting. The first leaves that appear are known as cotyledons, or seed leaves. These are followed by what are called true leaves. As soon as the true leaves enlarge,

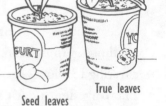

Seed leaves

True leaves

Chill Out!

Some herb seeds, such as echinacea, must undergo a period of cold before they will germinate. Satisfying a seed's chill requirement is called stratification. Norman Deno, chemistry professor emeritus from Pennsylvania State University, has a simple, space-saving approach to this process:

1. Dampen a heavy paper towel and fold it over to create a pocket.
2. Put the seeds in the pocket, and slip the towel and seeds into a small plastic bag, leaving it open slightly so moisture doesn't build up inside and rot the seeds.
3. Put the pocket in your refrigerator for three months. Remember to label it with the plant's name and the date you started the process, and to check the packet's moisture level periodically; the towel should be damp but not soaking wet.

you may transplant the seedlings to larger pots. From now on, once a week when you water, give them doses of water-soluble, organic fertilizer at one-quarter the recommended strength.

Hardening off. When it's time to move the young plants to their outdoor home, you'll need to harden them off for a week or so before transplanting them in the garden. This means taking them outdoors and putting them in a spot protected from direct sun, hard rain, or strong wind — under a shrub or a picnic table, for instance — then bringing them back in at night. Leave them out slightly longer each day. You should see them perking up and growing faster.

BUYING HEALTHY HERB PLANTS

If you don't have the time or space to start your seeds indoors, you can purchase your plants. In spring, you'll find greenhouses and tables at local garden centers laden with a tantalizing variety of young herb plants. The earlier you visit, the wider your choices are likely to be. Look for plump, bushy plants, not lean and lanky ones — herbs aren't fashion models! Choose young plants that are still putting their energy into leaves and roots, not ones in flower. Roots should not be growing through the pot's bottom. Look for leaves with deep, healthy-looking color, and check their undersides for any signs of discoloration or insects. If you find either of these, put the plant back. You don't want to transport diseases or pests to your garden.

EXPANDING YOUR GARDEN

Creating new plants by division, layering, and cuttings can be even easier than starting them from seed. Instead of a soft, vulnerable seedling, you will have a tough, hardened plant ready for the garden.

Division is the easiest method of propagating many clump-forming perennials, such as thyme or echinacea. And it's almost impossible to do it wrong. In spring or fall, dig up the clump and carefully break it into separate plants. For many herbs, you can do this with your hands, although you may need a serrated knife, saw, or hoe for tough, woody roots. Each section should have at least one stem as well as roots.

Replant the divisions at the same depth that the original clump was growing. If the herb has developed a bare, woody section in the center, throw away that part.

Layering is almost as easy, but requires a bit more patience. It's a good technique for herbs that are slightly woody but supple, such as sage, thyme, and lavender. Just pull down a side branch barely into the soil and secure it with a U-shaped wire. After several weeks, the branch will form roots where it is touching the soil. You'll know it's ready if it resists when you tug on it gently. You can then cut it from the mother herb and replant it.

Dividing echinacea

Layering sage

Mound layering. Some herbs, such as rosemary, sage, and lavender, tend to get bare and woody — just generally scruffy-looking — at the base as they mature. You can turn these old-timers into fresh young specimens through a technique called mound layering. In spring, mound garden soil over the base of the bare stems so that only the top of the herb is exposed, and keep the base covered throughout the season. By late summer or fall you should have new, rooted shoots that you can remove from the parent to pot or replant.

Mound-layering rosemary

Cuttings. The key to success with cuttings is keeping your tools and work area sterile, then creating a slightly humid environment that will encourage the cuttings to root. Use a soil-less medium that drains well. Some people use a mix of peat moss and sand, or even sand alone. Just vermiculite works fine for most herbaceous plants, but if the cuttings are at all heavy, they may fall over. Moisten the medium thoroughly before planting.

Most herbs are best propagated from what are called semi-ripe cuttings: new growth that has just started to harden. Fill a clean container with growing medium and make a hole in the center of the medium with a pencil. Using a sterilized knife or pruners, cut off a healthy shoot 3 to 5 inches long, with several leaves. Remove the last set of leaves on the bottom of the cutting. Dip the stem into rooting hormone (sold at garden centers), stick one third to one half of the cutting into the hole, and gently firm the medium around the stem. Bend a heavy wire, such as a coat hanger, into a hoop, push its ends into the pot, and drape plastic wrap or a plastic bag over this frame so that the plastic doesn't touch the cuttings. Put the pot in bright but indirect light. The cuttings should root in four to six weeks.

Keep It Clean

Use isopropyl alcohol (look for "70-percent solution" on the label) to sterilize all of the tools you use for plant propagation. Alcohol evaporates rapidly, so it does not need to be rinsed off, and it doesn't cause rust on your tools, as chlorine bleach solutions do.

Removing bottom set of leaves

Covering with plastic

CARING FOR YOUR HERBS

Once your herb garden is established, it won't require much maintenance. To make sure plants get the water and air they need, weed routinely, and water during long droughts.

FERTILIZING

Many traditional herbs are natural dieters. Rosemary, thyme, lavender, sage, and many other herbs that we use for both cooking and medicine come from Mediterranean regions where the soil is rocky and infertile. Growing in these harsh conditions actually encourages them to produce more of their essential oils. In fact, most herbs don't need, or even like, chemical fertilizer. High-nitrogen fertilizers produce soft, green growth that makes them more vulnerable to insects and disease. Just give them an annual top-dressing of compost or decomposed cow manure. You probably won't need to water them often, either, since their natural environment is on the dry side. Make sure the soil is well aerated (porous with gravel or fluffy organic material) so that it drains rapidly.

MULCHING AND DEADHEADING

Mulch will keep weeds to a minimum. Good mulches include compost, leaf mulch, and shredded bark, which all look nice and improve the soil as they decompose. You can help prevent root rot by keeping mulch away from the base of your herbs. And keep your eyes peeled for slugs and snails, which find heavy mulch a haven.

Some herbs are such ready self-sowers that they can be your herb garden's worst pests. These include angelica, fennel, feverfew, lemon balm and other mints, mullein, and St.-John's-wort. To keep these under control, deadhead flowers as they fade, before they have a chance to set seed.

Deadheading feverfew

HARVESTING YOUR HEALING HERBS

Harvesting your own herbs, like picking your own fruits and vegetables, is deeply rewarding. You'll feel a bit like strutting — after all, you've done such good work! At the same time, you'll want to fall on your knees to thank Mother Nature for her wonderful gift. Make your harvest a time of both celebration and leisurely reflection. Enjoy some quiet moments before the heat and hurry of the day, while you savor the plants' textures and keen aromas one more time.

HARVESTING AND DRYING EQUIPMENT

You'll enjoy the harvesting process most if you gather together all of your equipment beforehand. Keep your scissors and knife and some twine in a basket or container that fits into your gathering basket and you'll be all set to go when the crop is ready.

Sharp knife or scissors. If you break stems or use a dull knife, it batters the herb and hastens the loss of potency, so use a sharp tool to make clean cuts.

Flat-bottomed basket. Especially if you are collecting entire stems, this item will keep the plant from being crushed.

Paper bags. If you are collecting only leaves or flowers, paper bags work fine. Keep different herbs in separate bags.

Felt-tipped marker. Be sure to label all bags with a marker. Herbs become much less identifiable after they dry.

Twine, twist ties, or rubber bands. You need these to hang and dry your herbs. Preferences vary, but I prefer rubber bands, because they draw in as the herb stems dry and contract.

Coat hangers. You can attach several bundles of herbs to each hanger with wire or snap clothespins.

Small paper bags. Tie these around the heads of plants to catch their seeds for saving or preventing self-sowing.

Newspapers, paper towels, or cheesecloth. Use these to spread your herbs on and keep them clean.

Dehydrator. Sold for drying fruit and vegetables, these are quite efficient for herb drying as well.

WHEN TO HARVEST MEDICINAL HERBS

It's important to harvest medicinal herbs when their chemicals are most potent, and also to dry them quickly to preserve those all-important health benefits. Collect them on a dry day, in the morning just after the dew has dissipated. If you wait until too late in the day, hot sun can change the plants' chemistry. Light rain can spot them. Once you get to know your herbs well, you will develop an instinct about when they are ready for harvest. Their intense smells, plump healthy leaves, or just-opening flowers will almost seem to cry, "Pick me!" But the basic rules are easy to remember.

Leaves. Leaves, especially those of aromatic herbs, begin to lose their oils when their flowers bloom. Although you can start to harvest leaves earlier, plan to finish collecting all your medicinal foliage when you begin to see flower buds.

Flowers. Harvest flowers just as they start to open.

Seeds. Harvest seeds as they begin to turn brown. Don't let them get too ripe, or they will fall off! If you're afraid you may miss the moment, tie a bag around the seed heads to catch the seeds.

Berries. Gather berries when they are ripe (colored), but before they become soft. Throw away any that look moldy.

Roots. You can harvest roots in spring, before the herbs' leaves appear, or in fall, after the foliage has died back. At both times, the roots are

Early Harvests

You can harvest small amounts of many herbs throughout the growing season. In fact, some harvesting will encourage bushier growth. It's okay to collect up to half of the tops of annual and biennial herbs. After perennials have grown for a year, you can take as much as two-thirds of their top growth in late spring and another third in midsummer. Try to avoid harvesting much after that, because perennial plants need their leaves to continue manufacturing and storing energy for the winter.

Busting the Bite

Have you ever made pesto from basil after it flowered? If so, you'll remember that its sweet mintiness took on an unpleasant bite. That's what happens to the leaves of most aromatic herbs when they start to flower: At that point, the chemicals in their leaves change perceptibly. You can postpone the flowering process by pinching back buds periodically. Once the bloom phase is inevitable, however, finish your harvest for the season before the flowers develop fully.

more potent than during the rest of the year. Harvest the roots of biennials in the fall of their first year. It will be easiest to dig the roots after a light rain, when the ground is damp but not muddy. Cut them into sections or slice them right away, so that they can start drying.

Bark. If possible, trim off a mature branch and strip its bark. If you must take bark from the trunk because you can't reach a suitable branch, do so in the fall, when the tree's sap is down. Never strip bark all the way around the trunk of a tree; this is called girdling, and it will kill the tree. Instead, remove the bark carefully from one side. The tree will suffer less damage if you take bark from the north side, where the bark is often thicker because it gets less sun. Once you have removed the bark, strip off the rough outer layer and discard it. Place the inner layer on a tray or clean cloth in a warm, dry, well-ventilated spot.

DRYING YOUR HERBS

The traditional method of drying herbs is to tie them in bunches by their stems and hang them upside down in a warm (70 to 90°F), dry, well-ventilated place. They should be out of direct sun and away from any fumes, such as you might have in a basement or shed where you store paints and solvents or gasoline-powered equipment. An attic is ideal if it isn't too dusty. If seeds are still on the herbs, tie paper bags or cheesecloth over the heads to collect seeds as they fall. Use seeds medicinally, if appropriate, or plant for your next crop.

Stems. Magazines often show drying herbs displayed elegantly, suspended from wooden beams with twists of hemp. Other techniques may be less beautiful but more practical. A rubber band makes a good fastener, since it contracts as the herbs lose moisture and the stems shrink. Twist ties are good, too. You can fasten the bundles to a line with clothespins or, to save space, fasten several bunches of herbs to a clothes hanger. Depending on the size of your herbs, don't put more than three to six stems in a bundle. Keep the bundles 6 inches or more apart and away from walls.

Air-drying
herb bundles

Leaves and flowers. If you are drying smaller parts, such as individual leaves and flowers, spread them on newspapers or a clean cutting board. Better yet is a rack, such as a wooden dish drainer or an old window screen, that allows maximum air circulation. Lay a paper towel on top to keep the herbs from falling through. Don't use plastic, as water can condense on it. It's okay if the herbs touch each other, but be sure to stir them around occasionally to keep them exposed to air. Air-drying herbs can take up to two weeks, depending on the condition of the plants and the weather. They are dry enough to store when they are crisp to the touch.

Dehydrator. If you live in an area where it can be very humid at harvesttime, your herbs may become moldy before they have a chance to dry. A helpful device is a dehydrator — a small appliance sold for preparing

Go Easy on the Water

Don't wash your herbs unless they are excessively muddy, since this will slow the drying process and encourage mold. Roots will need cleaning, of course, but try not to soak them. You can get off much of the dirt with a toothbrush (unused!).

dried fruits and vegetables. In most models, a series of circular racks rotate while the base emits heat. You will probably need to put some cheesecloth on the racks to keep your herbs from falling through them. Leaves and flowers should dry in 4 to 10 hours; roots and berries may take up to 24 hours, depending on their size.

Microwave. If you don't have a dehydrator, a microwave is another option. A single layer of herbs, sandwiched between two paper towels, will often dry in 1 minute. If the herbs still aren't dry, reset the microwave and recheck the herbs at 30-second intervals. Because herbs vary substantially in the amount of moisture they contain, it's difficult to give precise timing, so be sure to watch them carefully so that they don't burn.

Conventional oven. Ovens rob many of the volatile oils from the herbs, but if you must use one, turn the oven to its lowest setting. Spread the herbs on a cookie sheet and check them periodically. The herbs can take a few hours to almost a day to dry, depending on how heavy and moist they are.

Freezer. You can freeze some herbs, primarily those with large, soft leaves, such as comfrey, lemon balm, mint, and parsley. Wash them, shake off the excess water, and put them in zip-top plastic bags in your freezer. They should be usable until the next herb-growing season. Use the same amount of frozen herbs as you would if they were air dried.

A Gardener's Guide to Medicinal Herbs

PLANT	PRIMARY MEDICINAL USE	MAXIMUM HEIGHT/SPREAD	PLANT TYPE	HARDINESS ZONE RANGE	LIGHT REQUIRED	SOIL
Angelica	Indigestion	8' / 4'	M	4–7	PS	Rich, moist
Black cohosh	Menopause	8' / 4'	P	3–7	PS/Sh	Rich, moist
Calendula	Skin injuries	2' / 1'	A	—	S	Average to rich
Catnip	Insomnia, indigestion	3' / 2'	P	3–9	S	Sandy
Chamomile, German	Insomnia, indigestion	3' / 1½'	A	—	S/PS	Sandy
Chamomile, Roman	Insomnia, indigestion	10" / 3'	P	5–9	S/PS	Rich, moist
Chaste tree	Menstrual problems, menopause	20' / 20'	Tree	7–9	S	Average to rich
Echinacea	Immunity booster	4' / 2'	P	3–8	S	Poor, acidic
Elderberry	Respiratory ailments	10' / 10'	Shrub	3–7	S/Sh	Average to rich
Evening primrose	Premenstrual syndrome	4' / 2'	P	4–10	S	Poor
Fennel	Indigestion	7' / 2'	P	5–9	S	Average, moist
Feverfew	Migraine headache	2' / 3'	P	5–7	S/PS	Average
Garlic	Cardiovascular health, infection	2' / 1'	(treat as annual)	5–9	S	Rich
Ginger	Motion sickness	3' / 2'	P	9–10	PS	Deep, rich
Hops	Sedative	25'	Vine	4–8	S	Rich
Horehound	Cough	1½' / 1½'	P	4–9	S/PS	Poor, dry
Hyssop	Cough	2' / 2'	P	4–9	S/Sh	Sandy
Lavender	Relaxant	3' / 2'	P	5–8	S	Gritty, alkaline

Chart Key:
A = Annual
B = Biennial
P = Perennial

M = Monocarp
S = Sun for 6 hours a day
Sh = Shade

PS = Partial shade; less than 6 hours of sun a day or filtered shade

HOW TO START, PROPAGATE	FEATURES	HARVEST
Sow seed outdoors in fall (don't cover seeds)	Dramatic form, short-lived	Leaves, stem, roots*
Sow seed outdoors in fall; root division	Fragrant white flower	Roots
Sow seed outdoors in spring, or indoors 4–6 weeks before last frost	Long-blooming yellow or orange flowers	Flowers, leaves
Sow seed outdoors in spring, or indoors 6–8 weeks before last frost	Fuzzy leaves	Leaves
Sow seed outdoors in spring	Daisylike flowers	Flowers
Buy plants in spring	Daisylike flowers	Flowers
Sow seed indoors or outdoors in spring or fall	Purple flowers, fragrant foliage	Seeds
Sow seed outdoors in fall, or seed outdoors in spring, but stratify seeds before planting; divide clumps	Pink, daisylike flowers	Roots second year
Plant fresh berries in spring; take softwood cuttings in midsummer	White flower clusters	Flowers**
Sow seed indoors in spring (don't keep too wet; soil should be 70–75°F; don't cover seed)	Yellow flowers in evening	Purchase commercial preparation
Sow seed outdoors in spring	Feathery foliage	Seeds, leaves
Sow seed outdoors 2 weeks before last frost, or, in North, indoors 8 weeks before last frost	Daisylike flowers	Leaves, flowers
Plant cloves in fall, 1–2" deep	Clusters of white flowers	Bulbs
Plant fresh roots any time	Subtropical	Roots
Buy plants in spring; divide strobiles (young shoots) in spring	Lobe-leaved	Fruits
Sow seed outdoors in spring or fall	Soft gray-green, fuzzy leaves and stems	Leaves, flowers
Sow seed outdoors in spring; take softwood cuttings; divide clumps	Blue flowers in late summer	Leaves, flowers
Buy plants in spring; take semi-hard cuttings in spring	Fragrant gray foliage, purple flowers	Leaves, flowers

*The fresh roots of angelica are toxic. Be sure to dry them thoroughly.
**Avoid using any uncooked parts of elderberry; the leaf bud, especially, is toxic.

Chart continued on page 98

PLANT	PRIMARY MEDICINAL USE	MAXIMUM HEIGHT/SPREAD	PLANT TYPE	HARDINESS ZONE RANGE	LIGHT REQUIRED	SOIL
Lemon balm	Sedative	2'/2'	P	5—9	S/PS	Average
Lovage	Fever, circulation	6'/3'	P	3—8	S/PS	Moist, rich
Meadowsweet	Pain relief	5'/3'	P	3—9	S/PS	Moist, alkaline
Mint	Indigestion	2'/4'	P	5—9	S/PS	Average, moist
Mullein	Respiratory ailments	6'/1½'	B	3—9	S	Sandy
Parsley	Urinary problems, bad breath	1'/2'	B	5—9	S/PS	Moist
Red pepper	Pain relief	3'/1½'	A	—	S	Sandy
Rosemary	Memory enhancement	1'/6'	P	8—10	S	Sandy
Sage	Memory enhancement	3'/3'	P	4—9	S	Average
St.-John's-wort	Mild depression	3½'/2'	P	3—8	S/Sh	Average
Thyme	Indigestion, cough	Variable	P	4—9	S	Sandy
Valerian	Sedative	5'/2'	P	4—8	S/PS	Rich, moist
Willow, white	Pain relief	80'/30'	Tree	4—9	S	Moist
Witch hazel	Aches, skin injuries	20'/20'	Shrub	4—8	S/PS	Rich, moist
Yarrow	Skin injuries	3'/2'	P	3—9	S	Average

Chart Key:
A = Annual
B = Biennial
P = Perennial

M = Monocarp
S = Sun for 6 hours a day
Sh = Shade

PS = Partial shade; less than 6 hours of sun a day or filtered shade

HOW TO START, PROPAGATE	FEATURES	HARVEST
Sow seed outdoors in spring, or indoors 8 weeks before last frost	Spreads readily	Leaves
Fresh seed in fall; divide roots in second year	Celery-like	Leaves, flowers, seeds
Buy plants any time; divide clumps in fall	Sweet-smelling, plume-like white flowers	Leaves, flowers
Buy plants in spring through early summer; divide roots in early spring (or, in South, in fall); root cuttings in water in spring and summer	Spreads rampantly	Leaves, flowers
Sow seed outdoors in spring	Flannel-leaved	Leaves, flowers, roots
Sow seed outdoors in spring, or indoors 4–6 weeks before last frost	Fine foliage	Leaves
Sow seed indoors 6 weeks before last frost	Bright fruits	Fruits
Buy plants after last frost	Blue flowers, fragrant leaves	Leaves
Freeze seed for 3 days, then plant frozen seed outdoors in spring 1–2 weeks before last frost, or indoors 8 weeks before last frost (don't cover seed); layer stems in late spring or early summer	Blue flowers, textured foliage	Leaves
Buy plants in spring; take softwood cuttings in late spring or early summer	Yellow flowers, invasive	Buy commercial preparation
Buy plants in spring or early summer; layer stems in late spring or early summer; take cuttings in spring; divide in spring or fall	Tiny, fragrant leaves	Leaves
Sow freshly gathered seed in fall; divide in fall	Fernlike leaves, fragant white flowers	Roots, second year
Buy plants in spring or summer; root cuttings in water any time	Spring catkins, spreading habit	Bark
Buy plants in spring	Fall or winter flowers	Leaves, bark, twigs
Sow seed outdoors in spring, or indoors 4–6 weeks before last frost	Yellow flowers	Flowers, leaves

STORING YOUR HERBS

Medicinal herbs have four enemies that can drain their healing power: light, heat, moisture, and air. When you store your herbs, the goal is to eliminate these factors as completely as possible. Use sterilized, airtight, ceramic, or dark-glass containers. Essential oils can dissipate through porous plastic containers. Containers should be filled to the top with the herbs you want to store. If you do have air space at the top, stuff in facial puffs or cotton balls. If the only airtight containers you can find are of clear glass, store them in a dark cupboard that you rarely open. Be sure that your storage shelves or cupboards aren't near a stove, radiator, or other heat source. Most herbs will retain their potency for only a year, so don't hoard your precious harvest beyond that. Make this a year of herbal adventure!

Check all of your stored herbs periodically to see if they are deteriorating. You'll know they have lost their effectiveness if they lose their characteristic aroma or crumble almost to a powder when you rub them between your fingers. Plants that contain mucilage, like marsh mallow, are especially prone to absorbing moisture.

Thinking Ahead

Make packets for herb seeds by recycling letter-size envelopes. Cut the envelopes in thirds and tape the open sides. If you have only a few seeds, you might want to cut the envelopes in quarters. The less air you allow in your packet, the fresher your seed will stay. Remember to label them with the herb name and date. Store the envelopes in a cool, dry place.

CHAPTER 5

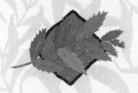

Symptoms
AND Remedies

U sing herbal remedies to prevent or treat injuries and illnesses is a little like planning a European vacation without a tour guide. You get to make your own choices — and natural ones at that. But it also means that you will need to do a little more homework so that you can make informed choices that will be right for you. This chapter provides you with all the basics about herbal remedies that can be used to cure symptoms of everyday or common ailments — safe doses, health cautions, and more. Whether you prefer to purchase ready-made herbal products or concoct your own homemade infusions, tinctures, and ointments, using herbs lets you be a more active participant in your health care.

CHOOSING THE BEST REMEDY

As you begin to explore herbal remedies, remember that, like synthetic drugs, herbs work because they contain effective — and sometimes very powerful — compounds. They may work more slowly than pharmaceuticals, but most herbs are also less likely to have side effects. For instance, if you take a decongestant for allergies, you probably expect a dry mouth or drowsiness as the price of feeling better. Instead, you could use stinging nettle to relieve your symptoms. It may take two days or so until you feel better, but on the other hand, you won't develop cotton mouth or fall asleep at your desk.

But just as we all react somewhat differently to prescription or over-the-counter medicines, we can expect to have different reactions to herbs. In addition, some herbs may be more readily available to us than others. Therefore, it's not practical for this book to lay out a single itinerary for every reader's exploration of herbal remedies. This section is set up to point you toward some initial good choices. For instance, for most symptoms covered in this chapter, you'll find one herb under the heading "Try This First." That's because it's the herb backed by the strongest research or evidence. But in each case, there are effective alternatives that you can use as well. You may have an uncomfortable reaction to one herb but not another, you may not have the first choice on hand the moment you need it, or you may simply not like the way the suggested herb tastes. So if the first choice isn't as effective for you as you'd like, try one of the other herbs described.

> ### When to Call the Doctor
>
> Remember, herbal medicines shouldn't take the place of a visit to your physician for chronic conditions or any condition that lasts for more than two or three days.

MAKE YOUR OWN REMEDIES OR BUY THEM?

You also have several choices about how and where to obtain most herbal remedies: You can grow your own herbs and prepare your own medicines, you can purchase dried herbs to make your remedies, or you can buy already-prepared medications.

Home-grown herbs. If you're a gardener, you'll probably want to grow as many medicinal herbs as possible, and after harvesting them, you may enjoy making most of your herbal preparations yourself. If you grow and harvest your own herbs, you know what is going into your herbal remedies and you know how they have been handled. You will also enjoy growing them just to get to know them, even if you can't grow enough for all your medicinal purposes. Being familiar with what the plant looks and smells like, from leafing out in spring through summer flowers and fall berries or seedpods, can help you feel more in tune with the herbal healing power that our ancestors recognized centuries ago.

Bulk herbs. You don't necessarily have to grow your herbs in order to make your own infusions, tinctures, salves, and even capsules. You can buy already dried "bulk herbs" from a health food store or supplier. Under each of the herbs in this chapter we suggest the form of home-made remedy (such as infusion or poultice) that is likely to be most convenient, and provide specific "recipes" and dosages to help you gain confidence and skill.

Bulk herbs, whether you grow them yourself or buy them, do have one disadvantage: Their strength and quality can vary a great deal, depending upon the amount of light and moisture the plant received, the fertility of its soil, whether it was harvested at the right time, and even its genetic makeup. Plus, bulk herbs stored improperly or for too long can lose potency. If you're not able to rely on their strength and quality, it's more difficult to determine the appropriate dosage.

Commercial preparations. Even if you don't have the space, time, or inclination to grow herbs or prepare your own medicines, you have a third way to enjoy the benefits of herbal remedies: Purchase them already prepared from a health food store or supplier. Not only is this often more convenient, but it has another advantage over using bulk herbs and making your own medicines: The potency of purchased remedies is standardized by the manufacturer, and therefore more reliable.

You should be able to find most of the herbs in this book in health food stores and, increasingly often, in grocery stores and pharmacies. You can also get them directly from a supplier (see Herbal Resources on page 146). Herbal medicines are usually packaged as tablets, capsules, or tinctures. Look for a package labeled "standardized herbal extract" or "guaranteed potency," which indicates that the active ingredient in the herb has been extracted and quantified. Although the labels aren't as informative as those on pharmaceuticals, those on standardized products tell you how many milligrams of extract are in each tablet, and whether the product contains fillers. In addition, the manufacturer recommends the appropriate dosage, based on that specific product. A common one for herbal capsules, for instance, is the advice to take "one to three a day with meals."

The best way to shop for commercially made herbal remedies is to compare two or three health food stores, organic groceries, or mail-order suppliers to see what they offer. Some may carry mostly capsules and tablets, while others offer a whole array of bulk herbs, tinctures, and essential oils. When you are just starting out, try to find products that contain an extract of a single herb, instead of something like "Mega-Super Energy Formula." That way you'll have a better idea of how individual herbs affect you.

Dosages for Homemade Herbal Remedies

If you're using herbs you've grown or homemade preparations, you may be uncertain how much to take. Because most herbs are so gentle, you can often be fairly relaxed about dosage, especially if you use a particular herb only occasionally. But because some herbs can have side effects if taken in large amounts or over extended periods, we have suggested dosages both in this chapter and in Chapter 3, beginning on page 27, based on what many expert herbalists recommend.

ACNE

During adolescence, hormonal swings cause sebaceous glands — which secrete an oil that lubricates hair follicles — to clog. This backup leads to a tiny rupture under the skin, which then becomes inflamed. Bacteria make redness and discomfort worse, so treat with antibacterial herbs.

TRY THIS FIRST

Tea tree. The essential oil made from the Australian tea tree (*Melaleuca alternifolia*) is one of the best bacteria fighters around. Use it directly on pimples. When trying it for the first time, you might want to dilute it, because it can irritate sensitive skin. Mix 1 part tea tree with 5 parts witch hazel and 5 parts rose water for a mixture that's astringent and smells good, too. Store in a cool, dark place.
Safety first. Do not take this or any essential oils internally.

Rosacea Is Red

During menopause, some women develop acne rosacea. It usually starts with a flushed-looking face, followed by pimple-like bumps. Buy calendula cream, or make a calendula tincture and mix it with an equal amount of rose water. Two drops of lavender oil will make the tincture even more soothing. Apply twice a day.

OTHER ACNE AIDS

Arnica. Arnica (*Arnica montana*) contains alcohol and other compounds that act as counterirritants, bringing blood to an injured area to speed healing. You can buy it as a cream or tincture, or make your own, using the flowers.
Safety first. Arnica is toxic, so never take it internally.
Calendula. Cleanse your face with a homemade or purchased cream containing this soothing antiseptic herb *(Calendula officinalis),* sometimes called pot marigold.
Garlic. Rub bacteria-fighting garlic cloves directly on pimples before bedtime. Or take purchased garlic tablets, or eat more raw garlic in your food. To counteract "garlic breath," eat sprigs of fresh parsley.

ALLERGIES

The word "allergy" covers a lot of ground, from an occasional annoying sneeze while you're cleaning house to life-threatening reactions to foods, drugs, plants, pets, and insect stings. If you know that your allergies are on the serious end of the scale, you should be under the regular care of a physician. Allergies are the result of the immune system's overreaction to the histamines that the body produces to fight potential invaders. We call substances that work against them antihistamines.

TRY THIS FIRST

Stinging nettle. This herb *(Urtica dioica)* won't beautify your perennial bed, but it has a huge number of fans among herbalists, for studies show that nettle contains a strong antihistamine. Buy stinging nettle capsules, and follow the label directions. Or, collect the leaves in early summer before the plant starts flowering. Wear gloves so you don't get stung by the toxin-filled hairs on the leaves; they will lose their sting once you dry or boil them. Herbalists recommend freezing the leaves to retain their antihistamine action. Make an infusion by steeping 2 teaspoons of the dried leaves in 1 cup of water. You can drink two cups a day.

Hay Fever Hazard

The periodic bouts of sneezing, watery eyes, runny nose, and cough known as hay fever are the result of seasonal allergic rhinitis. The culprit, or "invader," for the hay fever sufferer is wind-borne pollens. Tree pollen is the chief culprit in spring, grass pollen in summer, and ragweed pollen in fall.

ANOTHER ALLERGY REMEDY

Red pepper. Hot peppers can make you sniffle because they loosen mucus in your respiratory system. An article in the *Herb Quarterly* (Fall 1996) reports that they also desensitize mucous membranes to irritants and allergens, and curb inflammation as well. Add red pepper to your diet, or buy red pepper capsules and follow label directions.

ARTHRITIS

Arthritis affects 43 million Americans, including a quarter million children. There are over 100 different types, but the most common types are osteoarthritis, which affects joints and sometimes the spine, and rheumatoid arthritis, an autoimmune condition that can cause deformity.

TRY THIS FIRST

Ginger. This pleasant-tasting culinary root *(Zingiber officinale)* has anti-inflammatory properties. *Green Pharmacy* author James Duke reports on a study in India in which about 75 percent of those who took 1 to 3 teaspoons of ginger a day had less pain and swelling. After more than two years, they had suffered no side effects. Buy ginger capsules, and follow the directions on the label. Or grate the root and make a ginger decoction. You can drink up to 3 teaspoons a day.

Exercise for Arthritis

The Arthritis Foundation notes that exercise makes joints more stable because surrounding muscles are stronger. You'll develop more stamina and sleep better, too.

OTHER ARTHRITIS HELPERS

Red pepper. Red peppers *(Capsicum* species) contain an ingredient called capsaicin that stimulates the body's own painkillers and helps block pain perception. In addition to including more hot peppers in your diet, you can use them for a rejuvenating massage. Some nonprescription creams contain this ingredient (Zostrix is one brand name), or you can make your own ointments and creams using a red pepper infusion. Add 2 drops of lavender essential oil to your homemade salve or cream: Lavender's scent is relaxing, and its oil, like capsaicin, helps block pain perception.

Turmeric. This plant, *Curcuma longa,* also contains anti-inflammatory compounds. *Healing Herbs* author Michael Castleman recommends stirring 1 teaspoon of turmeric (available at grocery stores) into 1 cup of warm milk and drinking up to three cups a day.

Willow. Instead of taking daily doses of aspirin, use willow *(Salix species)*, which contains the same healing compound but is less likely to upset the stomach. Make a decoction by boiling about 1 teaspoon of the inner bark in 1 cup of water. You can drink up to three cups a day, with honey to mask bitterness. You can also buy willow bark in capsules; look for a standardized extract and follow the instructions on the label (usually two to three 380 mg capsules per day).

ASTHMA

Although many think of asthma as a childhood ailment, almost three times as many adults as children have this chronic disease. Airway passages get inflamed and swollen, sometimes after exercise or as a reaction to allergies, making it painful and hard to breathe. Anyone with asthma should be seeing a physician regularly, but there are a few herbs that may bring additional relief.

TRY THIS FIRST

Coffee and tea. Coffee and the widely available green and black teas (made from the leaves of a shrub, *Camellia sinensis)* contain stimulants that dilate bronchial tubes. Caffeinated colas and chocolate contain the same compounds. People with asthma have ended an attack by drinking a few cups of coffee when they've forgotten their medication.

OTHER HERBS FOR ASTHMA

Ginkgo. Popular as an asthma treatment in China, *Ginkgo biloba* interferes with a substance that causes spasms and constriction in the bronchial tubes. Buy a standardized product and follow label directions (typically, three 400 mg capsules a day).

Ginkgo

Stinging nettle. The antihistamines in this lowly weed can help people with asthma. Take nettle tablets according to label directions or make an infusion by drying the leaves and steeping 2 teaspoons in 1 cup of water. You can drink three to four cups a day.

BLADDER INFECTIONS

Women's anatomy makes them prone to infections — sometimes called cystitis or urinary tract infection (UTI) — that make urination painful. These infections are especially apt to flare up after sexual activity. Help prevent these infections by drinking a lot of water.

TRY THIS FIRST

Cranberry. Cranberry juice *(Vaccinium macrocarpon)* helps clear the urinary tract of germs. For prevention, you need to drink about 3 fluid ounces of juice a day. For treatment, increase that to 12 or more ounces.

OTHER HERBAL REMEDIES

Bearberry. This native ground cover *(Arctostaphylos uva-ursi)* is a cranberry relative that contains a diuretic and antibiotic substance. Make a decoction by boiling 1 teaspoon of bearberry leaves in 1 cup of water. Drink up to three cups a day for no more than a few days as a treatment. *Goldenrod.* The goldenrod species *Solidago virgaurea* is an aquaretic (an herb that helps you produce more urine by increasing blood flow in the kidneys). *Honest Herbal* author Varro Tyler calls it the most effective and safest aquaretic. Steep 1 or 2 teaspoons of the dried leaves in 1 cup of water. You can drink two cups of the infusion a day.

BRONCHITIS

Where the windpipe branches and heads for our lungs, it forms twin tubes called bronchi, and these branch again to become bronchioles. When these tubes become inflamed, we cough, wheeze, and, most tellingly, experience chest pain, so that it may hurt even to breathe. To treat bronchitis you need herbs that are expectorants (meaning that they will help you cough up the mucus in your lungs) and that are antibacterial, to help you fight the infection.

TRY THIS FIRST

Eucalyptus. This Australian tree herb *(Eucalyptus globulus)* is an excellent expectorant, reduces the spasms of coughs, and goes to work against bacteria that can cause bronchitis. Steep 1 teaspoon of dried leaves in 1 cup of water, and drink it three times a day. Breathing the vapor of steaming eucalyptus leaves can also be soothing.

Echinacea. As with other respiratory ailments, echinacea *(Echinacea angustifolia* and *E. purpurea)* may relieve bronchitis symptoms by beefing up your immune system. Buy echinacea tablets at your grocery or health food store, and use according to label directions.

Horehound. Horehound *(Marrubium vulgare)* contains marrubiin, an expectorant that's been used to treat coughs for 2,000 years. To make a tea, use ½ to 1 teaspoon of the dried herb per cup. Because this herb is so bitter, add 1 or 2 teaspoons of honey to each cup. You can also purchase horehound cough syrup or lozenges.

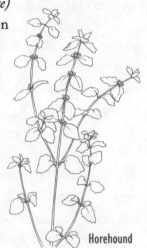
Horehound

Thyme. This culinary herb *(Thymus* species) is not merely an expectorant and antiseptic; it also helps relax the muscles of the respiratory tract. Use 2 teaspoons of dried leaves per cup to make a restorative and pleasant infusion.

BRUISES

Bruises, the visible result of tiny broken blood vessels under the skin, are sometimes just ugly, but they can also be painful.

Arnica. In addition to healing bruises, arnica *(Arnica montana)* helps reduce swelling. Buy a commercial cream containing this pain reliever, or make your own remedy by steeping 1 teaspoon of dried leaves in 1 cup of boiling water. Apply the infusion with a compress. *Safety first. Arnica is poisonous. Do not take it internally, and don't apply it if the skin is broken.*

OTHER BRUISE-BUSTERS

Comfrey. The roots and leaves of *Symphytum officinale* contain allantoin, a chemical that helps repair skin by encouraging cell division. It also reduces inflammation. Make a poultice of the leaves, or make an infusion and apply it with a compress.

Safety first. Do not use comfrey internally.

St.-John's-wort. Often used for curbing depression, St.-John's-wort *(Hypericum perforatum)* also reduces inflammation and fights bacteria. You can make your own ointment from St.-John's-wort leaves and flowers (the fresh flowering tops contain the most powerful healing components), or make a tincture or buy the standardized extract. Apply the tincture or extract directly to your injury, or dilute it with water and use with a compress. You can also apply the fresh, crushed flowers as a poultice.

Growing Comfrey

Comfrey grows 2 to 4 feet tall, with relatively small, bell-shaped flowers, usually purple, raspberry-pink, or white. It likes deep soil to accommodate its big taproot. Buy it as a root, and harvest the leaves before the flowers bloom in early summer.

BURNS AND SUNBURN

Most household burns, as well as sunburns, are first-degree burns, the least serious kind. When you blister, you have a second-degree burn, but if it's small enough to be covered with a first-aid strip, you can treat it at home. See the doctor for anything more serious.

TRY THIS FIRST

Aloe. The fresh gel from this spiky houseplant *(Aloe vera)* inhibits pain, promotes cell growth, and fights bacteria and fungus. Infection is the biggest danger when blisters form in second-degree burns. To use, cut off part of a leaf and press the exposed gel against the burned skin.

Calendula. This popular herb, *Calendula officinalis,* both soothes and reduces inflammation. Use a commercial cream containing calendula, or make your own salve, using a calendula infusion as described on page 20.

St.-John's-wort. A German study found that St.-John's-wort *(Hypericum perforatum)* healed first-degree burns in 48 hours. Buy or make a tincture and use it to whip up a homemade salve, or make an ointment following Method 2 on page 19.

CANKER SORES

Canker sores are painful, whitish ulcers that erupt inside the cheeks and lips. They can be triggered by acidic foods like dill pickles.

TRY THIS FIRST

Myrrh. Myrrh *(Commiphora myrrha)* gets top billing in the oral health category. Myrrh contains tannins, which contract damaged tissue, and it's antiseptic as well. Health food stores and suppliers offer capsules and tinctures. Apply a dab of either (if you're using capsules, open the capsule and pour out its powder) directly to the sore.

OTHER CANKER CURES

Goldenseal. Rinse your mouth with a decoction of this antiseptic and astringent herb *(Hydrastis canadensis),* using 1 teaspoon of dried root to 1 cup of water. You can sweeten its bitter taste.

Licorice. Licorice root *(Glycyrrhiza glabra)* contains tannins, mucilage, and healing compounds, and has a long history for treating the mucous membrane of the mouth and throat. Boil 1 teaspoon of the dried root in 1 pint of water for ½ hour, and use it as a mouthwash. Purchase the root from a health food store or supplier.

Goldenseal

Safety first. *People with heart problems or high blood pressure should use only deglycerized licorice.*

Sage. Like licorice, sage *(Salvia* species) contains tannins and has antibacterial properties. Make a tea with 2 teaspoons of dried herb to 1 cup of water and use as a gargle.

COLDS AND FLU

Even the mildest cold is enough to knock anyone off balance, and the accompanying muscle aches and exhaustion of flu can take us out of circulation for several days.

TRY THIS FIRST

Echinacea. Research shows that *Echinacea purpurea* multiplies and activates white blood cells that attack invaders. In clinical studies, echinacea extract reduced existing cold and flu symptoms, and it also helped prevent these infections in some people. Some herbalists advise taking it daily; others recommend that you take a standard dose only at the first sign of a cold or when you suspect you've been exposed. Buy tablets or capsules at a health food or grocery store, and follow label directions.

Echinacea

ANOTHER COLD COMFORT

Ginger. This tasty culinary root *(Zingiber officinale)* increases the body's ability to fight infection. Ginger also kills rhinoviruses, which cause colds, and reduces pain, fever, and coughing. Make a ginger tea with 2 teaspoons of grated root to 1 cup of water.

CONSTIPATION

You can generally avoid constipation if you follow good dietary practices: eating plenty of fresh fruits and vegetables and whole grains, and drinking a lot of water. At the first sign of constipation, take a high-fiber laxative herb, which absorbs water and forms a spongy mass. They don't work instantly, but you won't become dependent on them. Avoid herbs like cascara, which contain anthraquinones. Like most chemical laxatives, they can cause cramping and become habit-forming.

Psyllium. The seeds of *Plantago psyllium* and *P. ovata* are the primary ingredient in some commercial laxatives, such as Metamucil. They usually contain some sweetener or flavoring and are finely powdered. Run psyllium seed through an electric coffee grinder to make a more powdery substance.

More than a laxative, psyllium actually normalizes bowel function, since it can also work against diarrhea. You can take up to 3 tablespoons of seeds in 1 cup of water a day with meals; drink plenty of additional water to keep it moving through your system.

OTHER CONSTIPATION CURES

Flax. Flax seeds *(Linum usitatissimum)* swell when mixed with water. Take 1 to 3 tablespoons of ground seeds in water, and follow immediately with another 2 cups of water. Repeat this up to three times a day for acute constipation. For prevention, mix some flax with cereal, yogurts, or other breakfast foods.

Rhubarb. Like psyllium, rhubarb *(Rheum officinale)* can relieve either constipation or diarrhea. For constipation, take up to 1 teaspoon of the powdered root in 1 cup of water once a day. It may turn your urine red or bright yellow, but that's a normal side effect and not a cause to stop using the herb.

Safety first. Never use rhubarb leaves, which are poisonous. To avoid habit formation, don't use rhubarb for more than two weeks at a time.

Irritable Bowels

Irritable bowel syndrome is a chronic problem, sometimes caused by stress or an inability to tolerate certain foods, that causes swings between constipation and diarrhea. It may include other stomach problems like bloating and flatulence. Small daily doses of psyllium or flax can help bring things back to normal.

COUGHS

There are two types of coughs: a dry cough, often accompanied by a tickling sensation, and a wet cough that produces phlegm. Similarly, herbs can work two ways against cough, as antitussives and as expectorants. Many of these remedies are bitter, but you can flavor them with honey, which will also help soothe that irritating tickle.

ANTITUSSIVES

These herbs stimulate saliva and help suppress the cough reflex.

TRY THIS FIRST

Slippery elm. Recommended by the federal Food and Drug Administration (FDA), the inner bark of *Ulmus rubra* (formerly *U. fulva)* contains mucilage that soothes a sore throat. Collect the inner bark from one side (not all the way around, which can kill the tree). Make a decoction using 2 teaspoons of powdered bark per cup; drink up to three cups a day. Or buy lozenges, which deliver mucilage over a longer period.

OTHER COUGH SUPPRESSANTS

Marsh mallow. This pretty wetland native *(Althaea officinalis)* also contains mucilage, which will relieve that raw feeling. Use 2 teaspoons of the dried root in 1 cup of water.

Mullein. Verbascum thapsus is especially good for dry coughs. Use 2 teaspoons of dried flowers, leaves, or root per cup, and drink it up to three times a day.

Safety first. The seeds of mullein are toxic, so never take them internally.

EXPECTORANTS

These herbs thin mucus so that you can cough it up.

TRY THIS FIRST

Anise. Crush 1 teaspoon of *Pimpinella anisum* seeds into 1 cup boiling water and sip up to two cups a day.

Horehound. *(Marrubium vulgare)* contains marrubiin, which stimulates secretions of mucus in the bronchial tubes. Use about 1 teaspoon of dried leaves per cup, or purchase horehound lozenges.

Thyme. Garden thyme *(Thymus* species) is not merely an expectorant but also relaxes respiratory muscles so you won't experience so many racking spasms. Use 2 teaspoons of dried tops and flowers to make an infusion in 1 cup of water three times a day.

CUTS, SCRAPES, AND WOUNDS

When you get a minor skin wound, make cleaning it your first concern, before you apply any herb or other remedy. Many herbs are antiseptic, meaning that they stop the growth and reproduction of microorganisms such as bacteria, viruses, and fungi.

TRY THIS FIRST

Tea tree. The essential oil of this Australian tree *(Melaleuca alternifolia)* contains a powerful antibiotic, used for years by native Australians for all kinds of skin problems. Used "neat," tea tree oil may irritate your skin, so dilute 2 or 3 drops in 2 tablespoons of vegetable oil.

OTHER WOUND WONDERS

Aloe. The gel of this common houseplant *(Aloe vera)* stimulates cell growth, even when several layers of skin are injured. Use the gel fresh from the inner leaves.

Calendula. With 1 teaspoon or more of petals per cup of water, steep an infusion of *Calendula officinalis* to apply with a compress, or buy a commercial salve.

Comfrey. Comfrey *(Symphytum officinale)* stimulates healthy cell production, and stops inflammation. For skin wounds, use fresh, mature leaves as a poultice, applied directly to the injury. You can also find comfrey in commercial preparations for skin problems.

Safety first. Don't take comfrey internally.

Calendula

DEPRESSION

Severe depression is frightening and debilitating. If you have become despondent enough to miss work or avoid friends, or if you have even fleeting thoughts of suicide, you should contact a mental health professional. But if you have occasional bouts of the blues during which your energy flags, herbal remedies may help lift your spirits.

TRY THIS FIRST

St.-John's-wort. No other herb offers such a persuasive combination of long folk use and scientific evidence. In clinical studies of mildly or moderately depressed people, St.-John's-wort *(Hypericum perforatum)* outperformed many prescription antidepressants with few side effects. It probably works through a combination of compounds. Most mainstream physicians advise using the standardized extract, which is widely available in capsules.

Safety first. St.-John's-wort can cause supersensitivity to sunlight.

OTHER MOOD LIFTERS

Ginkgo. Depression in older people is sometimes caused by decreased blood flow to the brain, a condition that ginkgo *(Ginkgo biloba)* alleviates. Buy the standardized formula and follow label directions.

Licorice. Green Pharmacy author James Duke says that licorice *(Glycyrrhiza glabra)* contains more antidepressants than St.-John's-wort, and recommends adding some to herbal teas. Use ½ teaspoon of the powdered root per cup, and drink it twice a day.

Safety first. Long-term use of licorice can lead to headaches, water retention, loss of potassium, and high blood pressure.

Aroma-uppers

Essential oils of several plants can be mood brighteners. Here are some ideas from *The Essential Oils Book,* by Colleen K. Dodt:

- Keep rose water refrigerated in a bottle with a spray top to spritz on your face at the end of a tough day.
- Put a few drops of lavender oil on a tissue to carry with you.
- Add a few drops of clary sage to your herbal shampoo.

Siberian ginseng. Ginseng *(Eleutherococus senticosus)* not only contains antidepressants but also acts as an energizer and stress reducer. Buy a standardized extract and use it according to the label.

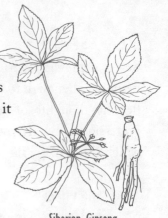

Siberian Ginseng

DIARRHEA

Even a brief bout of diarrhea can disrupt your life. A lot of things can cause diarrhea, and you should see a doctor if you have other symptoms with it or if it lasts more than a couple of days. But often we've just eaten something that "disagrees" with us, or picked up some unfriendly bacteria that have migrated to the intestines.

TRY THIS FIRST

Apple. Apples contain pectin, which coats the lining of the intestines and adds bulk to the stool. Eat two apples or a big helping of applesauce at the first sign of diarrhea.

The Importance of Water

Remember to drink a lot of water. It won't make your diarrhea worse, and severe diarrhea can quickly dehydrate you and make you seriously ill.

OTHER DIARRHEA STOPPERS

Blackberry, raspberry, or blueberry. The leaves of all three *(Rubus fruticosus, R. idaeus,* and *Vaccinium angustifolium)* contain high amounts of tannin, which "bind up" the intestinal lining and reduce inflammation there. Steep 2 teaspoons of the leaves in 1 cup of water. You can have up to six cups a day. Blackberry and raspberry leaves are often sold in bulk at health food stores; blueberry is available as tea and leaf extract.

Psyllium. Because these seeds *(Plantago psyllium* or *P. ovata)* work by absorbing water and making the stool soft and spongy, they also add bulk in a case of diarrhea. Take 1 teaspoonful three times a day with plenty of water.

Tea. Common black tea from the *Camellia sinensis* plant contains tannins that help bind and soothe the intestines. If diarrhea is a frequent problem, try drinking tea more regularly.

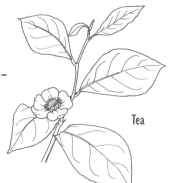

Tea

EARACHE

If you develop an earache as a symptom of a cold or other respiratory infection, you might want to fight the problem internally. Use pain relievers such as willow or immune-system boosters like echinacea, or make an infusion of one of the herbs that work for general respiratory problems, such as marsh mallow or elder. Or use one of the eardrops described below. (Never use eardrops unless your doctor has assured you that your eardrum has not been perforated. Otherwise, infection could lead to hearing loss.)

TRY THIS FIRST

Garlic. Garlic *(Allium sativum)* works internally or externally. Eat raw garlic for use as an antibiotic. Or, put a few drops of infused garlic oil (or garlic oil from purchased capsules) in the affected ear, or put the drops on a cotton ball and plug that in your ear.

Safety first. For ear drops, be sure to use homemade infused oil, not the powerful essential oil.

OTHER EARACHE EASERS

Eucalyptus. Inhale steam from hot water containing either leaves or a few drops of eucalyptus essential oil. Or massage a bit of the essential oil, diluted in vegetable oil, around the painful ear.

Goldenseal. To relieve middle ear pressure, buy goldenseal *(Hydrastis canadensis)* tablets and follow label directions.

Mullein. You can also make eardrops by steeping mullein flowers *(Verbascum thapsus)* in olive oil.

EYE PROBLEMS

We often strain our eyes by spending hours in front of computers and television screens. In addition, allergies as well as secondhand smoke and other air pollutants can make our eyes itch and burn.

TRY THIS FIRST

Eyebright. Eyebright *(Euphrasia officinalis)* has been used for centuries to help cure eye inflammations. If you have weepy eyes as the result of a cold or allergy, you can use it internally or externally. **Internally:** Make an infusion with ½ ounce of dried leaves in 1 pint of water, or buy capsules from your health food store and follow label directions. **Externally:** Steep 5 teaspoons of dried herb in 1 cup of distilled water; use as an eyewash no more than twice a day, or apply this infusion as a compress. Or, put 2 drops of eyebright tincture into an eyecup with distilled water.

Safety first. Strain any herb particles that could irritate your eyes, and sterilize the eyecup when you are done.

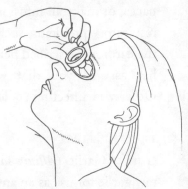
Using an eyecup

OTHER EYE SOOTHERS

Barberry. The powdered root bark of this garden shrub *(Berberis vulgaris)* contains an astringent alkaloid called berberine that constricts blood vessels and helps "get the red out" of bloodshot eyes. Boil ½ tea-

Not Pretty in Pinkeye

Pinkeye, or conjunctivitis, is a highly contagious infection of the conjunctiva, the outer skin layer of the eye. To treat it, wash your eyes with an infusion of eyebright, following one of the external-use procedures described under the eyebright entry above.

spoon of powdered bark (available at health food stores) in 1 cup of distilled water to make a decoction; strain carefully and use as an eyewash, or soak a cotton pad in the solution and apply as a compress.

Calendula. Use an infusion of pot marigold flowers *(Calendula officinalis)* on a compress to treat watery or irritated eyes.

Witch hazel. Soak cotton pads with witch hazel extract *(Hamamelis virginiana)* and place them on your closed eyes.

FATIGUE

In today's fast-paced world, we sometimes just try to do too much and need to slow down. Consider using some of the stress-busters under "Stress" on page 143. If you're eating a balanced diet, getting regular exercise, and sleeping 7 or 8 hours a night, you might want to get a full physical checkup to rule out any underlying illness.

TRY THIS FIRST

Ginseng. Ginseng reduces stress, sharpens mental acuity, and improves memory and the ability to concentrate. Asian ginseng may cause mild insomnia for frequent users, more than Siberian ginseng does. Buy a standardized extract and follow label directions.

OTHER PEPPER-UPPERS

Astragalus. The Chinese use the roots of *Astragalus membranaceus* (huang qi) as an energy booster. Studies show that it also has considerable ability to strengthen the immune system. Make a decoction by boiling 1 teaspoon of dried root in 1 cup of water, and drink it once a day. You can purchase dried root slices from health food stores.

Ginkgo. Ginkgo biloba stimulates blood flow to the brain, as well as to the heart. Buy the standardized extract and follow label directions.

Schisandra. In China and Japan, the dried fruits of *Schisandra chinensis* are a popular tonic, and research shows that the herb stimulates the nervous system and improves mental clarity. Look for a standardized extract at a health food store and follow label directions.

Safety first. Avoid schisandra if you have epilepsy or high blood pressure.

FEVER

Fevers above 103°F are not something for you to treat at home. Fevers lower than that are a signal that the body is at war against invading microorganisms. Still, fevers can make you miserable, so drink a lot of fluids and use some comforting herbs to ease the symptoms.

TRY THIS FIRST

Willow. Willow bark (*Salix* species) contains aspirin's active compound, but is gentler on the stomach. You might want to cover the bitter tang with ginger or cinnamon, which both have fever-relieving properties. Make a decoction by boiling 2 teaspoons of dried willow bark, which you can find at health food stores, in 1 cup of water.

OTHER FEVER BREAKERS

Ginger. Studies show that ginger *(Zingiber officinale)* reduces fever in small animals, and East Indian herbalists use it to lower body temperatures in humans. Make a decoction using 2 teaspoons of finely grated fresh gingerroot in 1 cup of water; drink one or two cups a day.

Meadowsweet. Benefit from salicin, the active ingredient in aspirin, by steeping 2 teaspoons of this towering perennial's flowers in 1 cup of water. Other ingredients in meadowsweet *(Filipendula ulmaria)* help make the salicin gentler to the stomach than aspirin.

GINGIVITIS

Gingivitis occurs when bacteria build up in the mouth and eat away at the gum tissue. First the gums bleed, then they begin pulling away from the teeth. Herbs with antiseptic properties kill those germs; those with tannins tighten soft gum tissues.

TRY THIS FIRST

Myrrh. Myrrh (a resin in *Commiphora* species) contains tannins and reduces inflammation. It is most effective as a tincture, available from health food stores or suppliers. Dilute 1 part tincture to 20 parts water, and use as a mouthwash.

Tooth Twigs

If you find yourself on a camping trip without a toothbrush, use the twigs from bay, eucalyptus, oak, fir, or juniper. All of them contain tannins that will tighten your gum tissue. Just break off a small branch, peel back the bark from the broken end, and use your fingernail or a small knife to "fuzz out" the fibers.

OTHER HERBAL GOODIES FOR GUMS

Licorice. Licorice *(Glycyrrhiza glabra)* soothes irritated mucous membranes and may slow plaque formation as well. Use it in a gargle with myrrh.

Sage. Sage *(Salvia officinalis)* leaves your teeth feeling smooth and your mouth refreshed. It also contains those all-important tannins and antiseptics. Drink it as an after-dinner tea.

HEADACHE

If headaches often keep you from working and playing at your best, you're hardly alone. It's estimated that 15 percent of Americans have headaches at least once a week, and as many as 12 percent of the population suffer from the excruciating, recurring type known as migraine. Three out of four people with migraines are women. A rarer type of chronic headache, called cluster headaches, usually affects men. Different herbs work for different types of headaches.

FOR COMMON HEADACHES

Ginkgo. *Green Pharmacy* author James Duke believes that ginkgo *(Ginkgo biloba)* may help headaches by increasing cerebral blood flow. Buy a standardized extract and follow directions on the label.

Lavender. Lavender (*Lavandula* species) contains substances that block the transmission of pain sensation. Dilute a few drops of essential oil in vegetable oil and massage it on your temples and neck.

Willow. Willow bark (*Salix* species) contains salicin, the ingredient first used to make aspirin. Make a decoction of 1 teaspoon of dried bark or powder (available in health food stores) per 1 cup of water. You can take three cups a day with honey or lemon.

Safety first. Don't take willow bark if aspirin bothers you.

FOR CLUSTER HEADACHES

Red pepper. Hot peppers (*Capsicum* species) are scientifically proven pain relievers, and the one herb that research has found to relieve cluster headaches. For prevention, try using more hot peppers in your cooking, but for relief of a headache, buy capsicum capsules.

Safety first. Remember to wash your hands after you handle red peppers so that you don't get the burning capsaicin in your eyes.

An Ounce of Prevention

Weather, food, and mood all can trigger headaches. Tension headaches, which usually occur as a steady, dull pain in the front of your head, may respond to relaxing herbs, such as chamomile, as well as regular exercise and yoga.

FOR MIGRAINE

Feverfew. In the 1980s, British scientists confirmed that *Tanacetum parthenium* helps reduce the number and severity of migraines, and stops the vomiting that sometimes accompanies them. As it's bitter and can cause mouth sores, take capsules; buy a standardized extract and follow label directions.

Feverfew

FOR SINUS HEADACHES

Eucalyptus. Sinus infections often cause headaches between the eyes and nose. Reach for eucalyptus (*Eucalyptus globulus*), a pain reliever and antiseptic. Dilute the essential oil in vegetable oil to massage into your forehead and the sides of your nose, or crush some leaves into a pan of hot water and inhale the steam.

HEMORRHOIDS

Hemorrhoids are swollen veins in the anus that become worse in people with chronic constipation. Many women develop them during pregnancy because of the pressure the baby creates.

TRY THIS FIRST

Psyllium. Having regular stools that are bulky yet soft will prevent hemorrhoids, and allow them to shrink and heal if you have them. Doctors recommend regular use of over-the-counter, psyllium-based *(Plantago psyllium* or *P. ovata)* laxatives, such as Metamucil.

OTHER HEMORRHOID HELPERS

Comfrey. This herb *(Symphytum officinale)* contains allantoin, which promotes new cell growth and fights inflammation. Make a decoction for a compress using 1 teaspoon of root boiled in 3 cups of water. Cut and powdered roots are available from health food stores.
Safety first. Don't use comfrey internally, since it may cause liver damage.
Mullein. Mullein *(Verbascum thapsus)* contains mucilage, which forms a soothing gel; tannins, which help shrink hemorrhoids; and some anti-inflammatory substances that help heal them. Buy dried flowers and leaves from health food stores and suppliers, and make an infusion to apply with a compress, or make a salve.
Witch hazel. Several commercial hemorrhoid preparations contain witch hazel *(Hamamelis virginiana).* An astringent, it also reduces inflammation, and research on animals shows that it constricts blood vessels as well. Make a decoction by boiling 1 teaspoon of powdered bark (available from health food stores) in 1 cup of water.

HIGH BLOOD PRESSURE

High blood pressure, or hypertension, is a serious condition that can eventually lead to heart attack or stroke. Because it sometimes has no symptoms, blood pressure readings are important. Normal pressure is 120/80. If your numbers are higher, a healthy diet can help bring them back down.

Garlic. As people age, their artery walls usually get thicker and harder, a condition called arteriosclerosis, or hardening of the arteries. High blood pressure and high cholesterol levels increase the risk of arteriosclerosis, but garlic combats both of these conditions. Eat one to three raw garlic cloves a day. Or, purchase garlic capsules; look for the standardized extract and follow the label instructions.

INDIGESTION AND HEARTBURN

Indigestion can be excess gas that bubbles up after you eat certain foods, food poisoning, or an infection like the so-called intestinal flu. Your tummy can be troubled when you're under stress or as a result of motion sickness. You may have stomach cramps or just feel queasy. One form of indigestion, heartburn, occurs when the "trapdoor" from the esophagus doesn't slam shut as it should.

TRY THIS FIRST

Peppermint. According to Varro Tyler, Purdue University's professor emeritus of pharmacognosy, this pleasant-tasting herb *(Mentha x piperita)* relieves gas, stops spasms in the upper digestive tract, stimulates bile flow, promotes stomach secretions, and kills bacteria. He recommends drinking a mint tea (1 tablespoon of dried leaves in ⅔ cup of water) three or four times a day. To extract even more benefit from mint's volatile oils, make a tincture with 7 ounces of dried mint in 1 liter of vodka. You can take up to 1 teaspoon of the tincture, three times a day.

Safety first. Give only a weak solution of peppermint tea to preschoolers, or they may choke on the menthol it contains.

OTHER STOMACH SOOTHERS

Chamomile. This herb *(Matricaria chamomilla* and *Chamaemelum nobile)* also acts against inflammation of the whole gastrointestinal tract. If you purchase it in bulk, look for whole flower heads without stems. Make or buy a tincture to capture more of the herb's active ingredients. You can take up to 3 teaspoons of tincture a day. An infusion is especially effective for heartburn. Use 2 to 3 heaping teaspoons of the dried herb to 1 cup of water. Heartburn usually occurs shortly after eating, so drink one cup after every meal.

Angelica. Germany's Commission E recommends *Angelica archangelica* for stomach cramps and indigestion because it relaxes the intestines. Boil 1 teaspoon of powdered dry root (available from health food stores and suppliers) in 1 cup of water for about 2 minutes. You can have up to two cups a day.

Safety first. The fresh roots are poisonous; dry them thoroughly. Angelica can increase sensitivity to sunlight. Pregnant women should avoid it, because it may stimulate uterine contractions.

Anise, caraway, and fennel. Available in most grocery stores, *Pimpinella anisum, Carum carvi,* and *Foeniculum vulgare* are among herbalists' favorite gas-reducing herbs. Just chew a few seeds before meals, or make infusions by crushing the seeds and steeping them. Use 1 teaspoon of the aniseed, and 2 teaspoons of caraway and fennel. You can drink three cups a day.

INSECT BITES AND STINGS

Mosquitoes, chiggers, and other bugs with a bite often seem determined to spoil summer fun. If you want to avoid chemical insect repellents, herbs can be the answer.

PREVENTING BITES

Several herbs can make insects keep their distance. Not only that, but these herbs smell good as well.

TRY THIS FIRST

Pennyroyal. You can rub the leaves of American pennyroyal *(Hedeoma pulegoides)* or European pennyroyal *(Mentha pulegium)* right on your skin. Pennyroyal is used in some commercial insect repellent products. Apply the strong essential oil only to clothing, not to your skin.
Safety first. Don't use pennyroyal, even externally, if you are pregnant. And don't use any essential oils internally.

OTHER BITE BLOCKERS

Citronella. Add 10 to 12 drops of citronella essential oil (*Cymbopogon* species) to 1 ounce of vegetable oil or baby oil, and rub it on your skin.
Mountain mint. Several species of *Pycnanthemum* are effective insect repellents. Keep several plants in your garden, and rub the leaves on your skin to repel insects.
Safety first. Don't use mountain mint, even externally, if you are pregnant.

Another Lemon-Flavored Repellent

Rub Lemongrass (*Cymbopogon citratus*) foliage directly on your skin for protection against insects. It grows in clumps 4 feet tall and about as wide. (Hardy only to Zone 9.)

RELIEF FROM ITCHING

If you do get stung, there are herbs that help take away the "ouch," as well as the itch.

TRY THIS FIRST

Aloe. Just as it soothes other skin irritations, the fresh gel from *Aloe vera* leaves relieves the itching and burning from bites.

OTHER ITCH EASERS

Calendula. Calendula, or pot marigold (*Calendula officinalis*), reduces inflammation, cools and soothes, and helps prevent infection. You can make your own calendula ointments and salves, but the commercial equivalents are easy to find in pharmacies and health food stores.

Garlic. Green Pharmacy author James Duke says garlic and onion *(Allium* species*)* contain enzymes that break down prostaglandins, which the body produces in response to pain. He advises mashing either garlic or onion bulbs to make a poultice for bites and stings.

Plantain. Colonists used plantain *(Plantago major)* to treat snake and insect bites. Crush some leaves and apply them directly to the sting.

INSOMNIA

When you don't fall asleep easily, or when you wake in the middle of the night, the next day can be a nightmare of poor concentration, shaky coordination, and nodding off at your desk. Drinking helpful herbs as warm fluids adds to the relaxing benefit.

TRY THIS FIRST

Valerian. Many herbalists consider valerian *(Valeriana officinalis)* the most effective of the sedative herbs. It's been used for centuries worldwide, and recent studies back up its reputation. Plus, it doesn't give the "hung-over" feeling you may get with commercial sleeping pills. Steep 1 teaspoon of dried root (available from health food stores or suppliers) in 1 cup of water before bedtime, or up to three times a day. The taste is bitter, so you may want to add honey or lemon, or purchase a tincture or capsules.

OTHER SLEEPYTIME HERBS

Catnip. The active compounds in *Nepeta cataria* are similar to those of valerian, but the effect is a bit milder. Catnip also tastes better than valerian, although not as good as other mints. Steep 2 teaspoons in 1 cup of water and drink before bedtime.

Chamomile. Scientists confirm that chamomile *(Matricaria chamomilla* and *Chamaemelum nobile)* contains sedative chemicals. Make your own infusion using 2 or 3 teaspoons of flowers to 1 cup of water. You can drink it three times a day.

Hops. Several Native American tribes used hop strobiles (the fruits of *Humulus lupulus)* to make sedatives. Recent research shows that when the strobiles are dried, they oxidize to form a substance that depresses the central nervous system. The German government's Commission E gives its seal of approval to hops for treating both anxiety and sleep disturbance. Steep 2 teaspoons of strobiles in 1 cup of water and drink it before bedtime. The taste is slightly bitter but not unpleasant.

Lavender. Commission E has pronounced this sweet-scented herb (*Lavandula* species) an official soporific, or sleepiness inducer. Studies with animals prove that lavender depresses the central nervous system. Lavender relaxes us through the sense of smell. Put a few drops of essential oil in a late-evening bath or on your pillow.

Passionflower. Studies on animals show that passionflower *(Passiflora incarnata)* makes them

Lavender

Getting More Sleep

If you haven't been sleeping well, consider making some changes in your lifestyle.

- Don't consume caffeinated beverages or chocolate after noon. Although caffeine affects people differently, its effects can last for many hours.
- Don't take daytime naps; they can take the edge off of sleepiness.
- Don't exercise in the evening. Exercise stimulates the body, making it more difficult to wind down and get to sleep.
- Don't consume alcoholic beverages. They can knock you out initially, but you will wake in the middle of the night when the effect wears off.
- Instead of a morning shower, take a warm bath with a few drops of lavender essential oil before you go to bed.

more "laid back"; scientists think several chemicals in it work in tandem as relaxants. Steep 1 or 2 teaspoons of the dried herb (available from health food stores or suppliers) in 1 cup of water, and drink it up to three times a day.

LIVER PROBLEMS

We rely on the liver to remove toxic substances from our bodies, and sometimes we work it too hard. Most liver damage is caused by excessive alcohol consumption, but the liver can also be damaged by medications, food additives, and air pollutants. Hepatitis, an inflammation of the liver caused by many things, including viruses, strikes more than a quarter million Americans a year. It should be treated by a physician, but herbal medicines may help speed recovery.

TRY THIS FIRST

Milk thistle. A lot of impressive research on this thistle *(Silybum marianum)* shows that it not only protects the liver from damage, but may even help regenerate cells after they are damaged from toxins or disease. Milk thistle capsules are available from health food stores or suppliers; follow the advice on the label. Or, make your own infusion by steeping 1 teaspoon of crushed seeds in ½ cup of water, and drink up to 1½ cups a day.

OTHER LIVER CLEANSERS

Dandelion. Eat dandelion greens, fresh or steamed, or make an infusion. Steep about ½ ounce of dried leaves or 2 to 3 teaspoons of powdered root per cup of water. Use up to three cups a day.

Licorice. Licorice *(Glycyrrhiza glabra)* contains a compound called glycyrrhizin that may help protect the liver. Asian doctors use licorice to treat liver problems, particularly hepatitis. Buy powdered licorice root or extract from a health food store, and follow label directions.

Safety first. If you are under a doctor's care for hepatitis, be sure to consult with him or her before using this or any other herbs for supplementary treatment. People with heart problems or high blood pressure should take only deglycerized licorice (available from health food stores or suppliers). Glycyrrhizin can cause weakness and swelling of the face and ankles.

MEMORY LOSS

All of us dread the detriments of aging, especially the loss of our mental abilities. Scientists continue to look for ways of treating the serious memory loss of Alzheimer's disease, but several herbs may help prevent less profound mental difficulties.

TRY THIS FIRST

Ginkgo. One cause of short-term memory loss is cerebrovascular disease, caused by abnormal blood flow to the brain as a result of arteries clogged by atherosclerosis. A ginkgo leaf extract *(Ginkgo biloba)* called GBE strengthens blood capillaries, makes blood more fluid, and increases blood circulation in the brain. It even helps the brain tolerate hypoxia, a reduced oxygen supply that occurs from sluggish blood flow. Look for a standardized extract and follow label directions.

OTHER MEMORY REMEDIATORS

Ginseng. Ginseng *(Panax quinquefolius, P. ginseng,* and *Eleutherococus senticosus)* seems to enhance memory. Herbalists recommend it to help older people concentrate better and react more quickly. Most research has been done on the Korean species, but Siberian ginseng seems to have most of the same properties and costs about one-tenth as much. Look for capsules from health food stores or suppliers.

Rosemary. Long known as the herb of remembrance, rosemary *(Rosmarinus officinalis)* contains antioxidants — security guards against free radicals, the oxygen molecules that speed aging. Use 1 teaspoon of dried rosemary to make a cup of daily remembrance tea.

MENOPAUSE

When women around the age of 50 start having hot flashes, vaginal dryness, night sweats, and mood changes, they can take hormone replacement therapy (HRT), which lessens bone loss (osteoporosis) and possibly wards off heart disease. But HRT can also increase the risk of breast cancer and cause other unpleasant side effects. Many herbs can decrease the woes of menopause, without side effects. But don't take them in combination with HRT without consulting your physician.

TRY THIS FIRST

Black cohosh. Most experts agree that this native plant *(Cimicifuga racemosa)*, also called snakeroot, takes the edge off menopausal symptoms. Some recommend it for anxiety, irritability, and sleeplessness. Other research shows that it contains estrogen-like compounds that reduce hot flashes and depression. It may also relieve vaginal dryness. Decoct ½ teaspoon of powdered root (from health food stores) in 1 cup of water, and sip 2 or 3 tablespoons at a time during the day.

Safety first. *Don't take it if you have any heart problems, if you take medication or herbs for high blood pressure, or if you notice any side effects, such as lightheadedness or stomach upset. Don't take it for longer than six months without a break. And, don't take it if you might be pregnant.*

OTHER MENOPAUSE MANAGERS

Chaste tree. Most studies of *Vitex agnus-castus* relate to its ability to alleviate premenstrual syndrome (PMS). But it may also reduce similar distress during menopause. The standard daily dose is 20 to 40 mg (about ⅛ teaspoon of the crushed, dried berries, available from health food stores and suppliers). Boil them in 1 cup of water.

Chinese angelica. The Chinese herb dong quai *(Angelica polymorpha* var. *sinensis)* may also make menopause more bearable. Boil 2 teaspoons of powdered root (available at health food stores) in 1 cup of water for 2 minutes. Drink up to two cups a day.

Safety first. *Be sure to use the dried root; the fresh root is poisonous. Using angelica regularly may make you supersensitive to sunlight.*

• For vaginal dryness, apply vitamin E or comfrey ointment.
• For mild depression, try St.-John's-wort, licorice, ginkgo, or Siberian ginseng.
• For overall symptom reduction, include more beans and soy products like tofu in your diet. These can help normalize estrogen levels.

To prevent osteoporosis (a condition of aging that makes bones brittle and fractures more likely):
• Load up on low-fat varieties of yogurt, cottage cheese, and milk.
• Take a calcium supplement.
• Get regular weight-bearing exercise, including aerobic exercises and weight lifting.

Sage. This culinary herb helps combat hot flashes and night sweats. Simmer 1 or 2 teaspoons in 1 cup of water, and drink it during the day for hot flashes and before bedtime for night sweats. You can have three cups a day. It may increase vaginal dryness.

MENSTRUAL PROBLEMS

Countless herbs have been tried in the past for "women's problems," and a few have stood the test of time. Many of these contain some substances similar to estrogen. If you take birth control pills, don't take any estrogen-like herbs without discussing them with your doctor. And don't use any of these herbs if you think you may be pregnant.

TRY THIS FIRST

Chaste tree. Research shows that the dried berry of *Vitex agnus-castus* can realign irregular periods and help balance "raging hormones" by lowering the secretion of estrogen. In one study, women found it more helpful than vitamin B_6 in easing premenstrual syndrome (PMS), that medley of bloating, bad mood, and breast tenderness. And *Vitex* contains phytoestrogens, which can help reduce the risk of breast cancer. The standard dose is ½ teaspoon of the crushed seeds, boiled in 1 cup of water. Drink one cup a day starting about a week before your period. *Safety first.* Women who are depressed during PMS should avoid chasteberry, which can raise levels of the hormones that lead to depression.

OTHER MENSTRUAL MODERATORS

Burdock. This common weed, *Arctium lappa,* contains estrogen-like compounds. It's also a diuretic, so it flushes out excess water that causes uncomfortable pre-period symptoms like bloating and breast tenderness. Steep 1 teaspoon of dried roots (available from health food stores) in 2 cups of water for ½ hour, and drink one or two cups a day.

Evening primrose. Native American women chewed the seeds of this night-blooming perennial *(Oenothera biennis)* to relieve menstrual discomfort. Buy capsules of the seed oil; the usual recommended dose is three to six capsules a day.

Feverfew. An antispasmodic, feverfew *(Tanacetum parthenium)* relaxes the uterus and neutralizes prostaglandins that may make menstrual periods painful. To ease cramps or bring on delayed menstruation, steep ½ teaspoon of the dried leaves in 1 cup of water, and drink two cups a day.

Yarrow. Another antispasmodic, yarrow *(Achillea millefolium)* may ease cramps and work as a mild tranquilizer. Use 1 or 2 teaspoons of dried leaves or flowers in 1 cup of water, and drink three cups a day. Yarrow may turn your urine brown, but this is not harmful.

Treating Your PMS Symptoms

- For depression, try one of the herbs recommended under "Depression" on page 117.
- For edginess and irritability, try a calming herb like lemon balm, mint, or chamomile.
- For bloating and breast tenderness, drink more water and munch on parsley, which is a diuretic.

Nausea and Motion Sickness

Mild food poisoning, motion sickness, morning sickness, consuming too much alcohol, and stress can all cause a queasy stomach. If you have other symptoms or your nausea lasts more than a day, see your doctor. For a garden-variety upset tummy, give these herbs a try.

TRY THIS FIRST

Ginger. Delicious and gentle, ginger *(Zingiber officinale)* is most herbalists' first choice for nausea of any kind. If you have motion sickness, ginger also helps reduce dizziness. You can chew on the root, buy capsules from a health food store or supplier, or make a decoction with 2 teaspoons of powdered or grated root in 1 cup of boiling water.

OTHER TUMMY PACIFIERS

Mint. Menthol is the compound in peppermint *(Mentha x piperita)* and spearmint *(M. spicata)* that soothes sour stomachs. Steep 1 or 2 teaspoons dried leaves in 1 cup water, and drink three cups a day.
Safety first. If you have morning sickness, drink only diluted mint tea, and none at all if you have a history of miscarriage.
Raspberry. Steep 1 teaspoon of the dried leaf *(Rubus idaeus)* in 1 cup of water, and drink two cups a day.

Pain

Pain may be nature's way of telling us something's wrong. Sometimes it stems from an injury that takes days or weeks to heal; sometimes it's from a chronic problem like arthritis that flares up and then subsides. Don't try self-diagnosing the reason for your pain. But once you're sure of the cause, some herbs may help to ease it.

TRY THIS FIRST

Red pepper. Peppers *(Capsicum* species) contain capsaicin, a substance that combats pain in two ways. If you ingest peppers, it rouses endorphins, the body's natural painkillers. If you rub it on your skin, it interferes with pain transmission. Make a decoction with ¼ to 1 teaspoon of dried red pepper in a cup of water, or purchase capsules. For external use, use commercial skin creams with capsaicin, or add a cayenne decoction to your favorite cream or salve, and massage the painful area.

MORE PAIN STOPPERS

Meadowsweet. Filipendula ulmaria contains salicin, and it's even milder than willow, in which this pain-relieving chemical was first discovered. Steep 1 or 2 teaspoons of the dried leaves and flowers in 1 cup of water, and drink up to three cups a day.
Safety first. Don't use meadowsweet if you have problems taking aspirin.
Willow. Chemists developed aspirin from salicin, the active compound in willow *(Salix* species). Willow bark is much gentler than aspirin, but species differ in the amount of salicin they contain. The species most commonly sold is white willow *(S. alba)*. Simmer 1 to 5 teaspoons of dried inner bark per cup of water for ½ hour. Drink up to three cups a day.
Safety first. Don't use willow bark if you have problems taking aspirin.

POISON IVY, POISON OAK, AND POISON SUMAC

Eighty-five percent of the population have a severe allergic reaction to urushiol, an oil found in the leaves, stems, and roots of poison ivy, oak, and sumac. The itchy, blistery rash usually disappears in about two weeks. But in the meantime, you'll try just about anything to stop the itching.

TRY THIS FIRST

Plantain. Once your skin has erupted with bumps and blisters, make a poultice of plantain leaves *(Plantago major)* to soothe the itch.

ANOTHER ANTI-ITCHER

Aloe. Aloe vera is soothingly cool and it also prevents infection. Slice the leaf lengthwise, and lay the leaf on the irritated skin.

PROSTATE ENLARGEMENT

By the time men hit their half-century mark, 50 percent of them have an enlarged prostate, the little gland that produces seminal fluid. Located at the base of the urethra (the tube that carries urine out of the body), an enlarged prostate makes it difficult to urinate.

TRY THIS FIRST

Saw palmetto. The reason the prostate gland enlarges is that testosterone is converted into another form that makes the gland's cells multiply too fast. Saw palmetto *(Serenoa repens),* listed by the FDA as beneficial, slows this process. Look for capsules where you buy herbs and follow the directions on the label.

ANOTHER PROSTATE HERB

Stinging nettle. In one well-done study, stinging nettle *(Urtica dioica)* helped reduce the need for nighttime urination. Scientists think that, like saw palmetto, nettle keeps testosterone from being changed into its hyperactive form. Try 2 teaspoons of the dried leaves steeped in 1 cup of water, once a day. Or buy capsules and follow label directions.

SEXUAL DRIVE, HERS

Loss of libido can be distressing to those who have enjoyed sex in the past — especially if they're in an otherwise happy relationship with someone whose passions are still in high gear.

TRY THIS FIRST

Chinese angelica. Chinese women take dong quai *(Angelica polymorpha* var. *sinensis)* for such problems as painful or irregular menstruation and PMS. Use 1 tablespoon of powdered root (available from health food stores and suppliers) in 1 pint of water and boil it for ½ hour. You can take two cups a day.

Safety first. Don't use Chinese angelica if you are pregnant; it can cause uterine contractions.

Ginseng. Native American tribes used our native ginseng as an aphrodisiac. Korean ginseng *(Panax ginseng)* has always had a reputation for increasing libido in men, and now there are reports that it works in women as well. Buy capsules and follow label directions.

Why Has the Fire Gone Out?

Men become impotent and women lose their desire to have sex for similar reasons: physical illness, depression, fatigue, use of prescription drugs or alcohol, problems within a relationship. If none of these seems to fit you, consider talking to your doctor to make sure you can rule out any underlying physical cause before you turn to using herbs.

SEXUAL DRIVE, HIS

With Viagra available, why should you consider herbs to treat impotence? Viagra is expensive, and if yours is a mild or sporadically occurring problem, you might want to try a more natural approach first.

Ginkgo. Ginkgo biloba stimulates blood flow, which is crucial to penile erection. In tests on men whose atherosclerosis blocked blood vessels to the penis, researchers found that half who took ginkgo achieved erections. The subjects took 60 mg of extract daily.

Safety first. If you use this herb over a period of months, it's best to consult your physician.

SKIN RASHES AND DRYNESS

Allergic reactions to food, medicine, skin lotion, or pets, as well as extreme stress, can all trigger rashes. Dry skin is another common problem, often worsened in winter when heated, unhumidified indoor air makes us itch and peel. Eczema is a more miserable condition in which inflamed skin becomes red and forms scaly patches.

TRY THIS FIRST

Calendula. Pot marigold *(Calendula officinalis)* goes to work against inflammation and infection. Buy a ready-made cream; make an infusion by steeping 2 teaspoons of the flowers in 1 cup of water and apply it with a compress; or add the dried flowers to your favorite skin cream.

MORE SKIN SALVATION

Stinging nettle. If your itch is allergy related, take stinging nettle *(Urtica dioica)* capsules, available from health food stores or suppliers, or make an infusion with 1 or 2 teaspoons of dried nettle leaves or root in 1 cup of water. You can have two cups a day.

Safety first. Wear gloves and long sleeves if you harvest your own nettle.

Ivy. The leaves of common English ivy *(Hedera helix)* contain saponins, which get soapy when they're mixed with water. Crush a handful of leaves to make a poultice.

Johnny-Jump-Up

The flowers and leaves of Johnny-jump-up *(Viola tricolor)*, also called heart's ease, contain mucilage and saponins, which form a soothing lather for itchy skin when they're mixed with water. You can also drink a heart's-ease infusion for eczema, impetigo, and other skin irritations. To treat hives, try steeping equal parts of heart's ease (available from health food stores and suppliers) and calendula (about 2 teaspoons of each) in 1 pint of water, and sip it throughout the day.

Plantain. Plantago major is a mucilage-filled plant that forms a soothing emollient gel in water; it also fights inflammation and bacteria. Crush the leaves and apply them as a poultice.

Gotu kola. In a cream, this herb *(Centella asiatica)* from India helps relieve the painful, scaly welts of psoriasis and promotes blood circulation, which can speed healing. Add the commercial tincture to an ointment or salve. Or add ½ teaspoon of the dried leaves to 1 cup of water, and apply to skin as a compress.

SORE THROAT

Sore throats often accompany colds, flu, and allergy attacks. Herbs containing a lot of mucilage soothe a sore throat's scratchiness and may help with laryngitis, too.

TRY THIS FIRST

Licorice. Licorice *(Glycyrrhiza glabra)* roots are rich in mucilage, as well as glycyrrhizin, which suppresses coughs that make a sore throat even more agonizing. Make a licorice decoction by boiling about ½ teaspoon of powdered root per cup of water. Gargle it, or take a whole day to drink a cup or two, sipping a little at a time.

Safety first. Stop using licorice if you experience weakness, headaches, or swelling. If you have high blood pressure or heart disease, use only deglycerized licorice.

OTHER THROAT SOOTHERS

Horehound. This old-time remedy *(Marrubium vulgare)* is a popular cough medicine, but its mucilage also soothes sore throats. Steep 1 teaspoon of leaves and flowers in 1 cup of water, and sip up to three cups a day. You can also find horehound lozenges wherever cold and flu remedies are sold.

Marsh mallow. The root of this wetland shrub *(Althaea officinalis)* contains mucilage and has anti-inflammatory powers. Boil about 1 teaspoon of the dried root (available from health food stores and suppliers) in 1 cup of water, and drink, or sip, up to three cups a day.

Mullein. Like other herbs used for sore throat, mullein *(Verbascum thapsus)* contains mucilage, and bracing tannins as well. You can use 1 or 2 teaspoons of dried leaves, roots, and flowers, per cup of water. Flavor it with some honey, lemon, or licorice.

Safety first. Mullein seeds are poisonous.

Slippery elm. The powdered bark of this tree *(Ulmus rubra)* contains soothing mucilage as well as antiseptic chemicals. Make a decoction by simmering 2 teaspoons of the powdered bark in 1 cup of water for about 15 minutes. Sip a bit at a time, taking up to three cups a day.

STRAINS AND SPRAINS

You don't have to be an athlete to be injured and out of action. It's easy to wrench a shoulder gardening or twist an ankle on an errant toy. Herbs can reduce inflammation or swelling.

TRY THIS FIRST

Red pepper. Rubbing red pepper *(Capsicum* species) on your skin causes irritation that may distract you from deeper pain while it stimulates blood flow, which can speed healing. Mix 1 teaspoon of powdered cayenne in ½ cup of vegetable oil (use more or less depending on your skin's sensitivity).

Safety first. Wash your hands thoroughly after you handle peppers so you don't get their hot capsaicin in your eyes.

OTHER INJURY HEALERS

Comfrey. Comfrey *(Symphytum officinale)* works against pain, swelling, and inflammation. Make a poultice with dried powder, using just enough water to make a paste, or add it to a skin lotion.

Safety first. Comfrey is linked to liver cancer; don't use it internally.

Pineapple. Green Pharmacy author James Duke recommends this tropical fruit, containing the enzyme bromelain. Pineapple *(Ananas comosus)* reduces inflammation and helps reduce swelling and pain. To offset muscle and joint pain, eat pineapple or get bromelain capsules and tablets from health food stores or suppliers; follow label directions.

Turmeric. This culinary herb *(Curcuma longa)* lessens inflammation whether you take it internally or use it externally. Researchers have found that juice from its root reduces swelling, and in a dry powder form it relieves arthritis pain. Look for capsules containing the active ingredient, curcumin, in health food stores or suppliers' catalogs.

STRESS

Feeling anxious, overworked, tense, and jittery isn't just unpleasant; it can also erupt in all sorts of physical problems, including upset stomach, headache, and hives, and it can even shorten your life span.

TRY THIS FIRST

Valerian. Most herbalists regard valerian *(Valeriana officinalis)* as the strongest of the sedative herbs. In Germany it's an ingredient in commercial tranquilizers, and it's endorsed by our own FDA. Studies with animals show that it may help lower blood pressure. Steep 2 teaspoons of the powdered root (available from health food stores and suppliers) in 1 cup of water.

OTHER PACIFYING PLANTS

Catnip. *Nepeta cataria* has the opposite effect on humans than it does on cats. Steep 2 teaspoons of the dried leaves in 1 cup of water, and drink it three times a day.

Passionflower. Michael and Janet Weiner, authors of *Herbs That Heal,* say this native vine *(Passiflora incarnata)* "may be our best tranquilizer yet." It relieves muscle tension and fatigue, too. Recent research on one species indicates that it may lift depression as well, so it may be an effective overall mood leveler. Use 1 teaspoon of dried leaves (available from health food stores or suppliers) to make a cup of tea, and drink it three times a day when the world is getting you down.

Skullcap. Chinese studies have shown that *Scutellaria lateriflora* depresses the central nervous system, the sign of an effective sedative. According to a study in Japan, it also increases the level of good cholesterol, thus reducing the likelihood of heart attack and stroke. Steep

1 or 2 teaspoons dried leaves in 1 cup of water up to three cups a day. Purchase skullcap in bulk herb, as tea, or in capsules or tinctures.

Safety first. Don't use skullcap if you're pregnant.

Lemon balm, chamomile, hops, and lavender. All of these herbs *(Melissa officinalis, Matricaria chamomilla* and *Chamaemelum nobile, Humulus lupulus,* and *Lavandula* species) can help calm you down. Use the amounts recommended for these herbs under "Insomnia" on page 129, drinking them during the day when you feel tense.

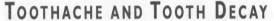

Hops

TOOTHACHE AND TOOTH DECAY

One important component of good health care is, of course, visiting your dentist twice a year. But if you develop an occasional toothache, herbs can relieve your agony.

FOR TOOTHACHE

Clove. Some dentists use this spice (the dried, unopened flower bud of a tropical evergreen tree, *Syzygium aromaticum*) to numb patients' mouths. It's antiseptic, too, and you'll find it in commercial products for toothaches. Apply 2 or 3 drops of clove essential oil around your aching tooth while you wait to see the dentist. For a mouthwash, simmer 1 teaspoon of powdered cloves in 1 cup of water for 15 minutes.

Safety first. Clove oil, like all essential oils, should not be ingested.

Ginger. This hot, sweet root *(Zingiber officinale)* helps by rushing blood to the spot to speed healing. Try pressing some of the fresh root (available at the grocery store) against your tooth, or make a paste of powdered ginger and apply it with your finger.

FOR TOOTH DECAY

Tea. Common tea, made from the leaves of *Camellia sinensis,* is full of cavity-fighting fluoride. Tea also contains tannins and other substances that do a job on decay-causing bacteria.

WEIGHT MANAGEMENT

Americans are obsessed with weight, yet resolution often crumbles when the dessert tray comes around. Some herbs might help you lighten the load, but they're certainly not a replacement for consuming fewer calories with less fat and more fiber, and exercising regularly.

Psyllium. Because plantain seeds swell when they get wet, they might help you feel less hungry. In addition, when partially digested food passes through the intestine, psyllium reduces the amount the body absorbs. Mix 1 heaping teaspoon in a glass of water ½ hour before mealtime, then drink another glass of water.

Red pepper. Research shows that red pepper (*Capsicum* species) can raise metabolic rates as much as 25 percent. *Green Pharmacy* author James Duke suggests eating 2 teaspoons of hot sauce with a meal. Red pepper capsules are available if you'd prefer to take your "heat" in a blander manner.

Stimulating Your Appetite

Lack of appetite can be a life-or-death issue. The herbs known as bitters may help by stimulating saliva flow and stomach secretions, so you feel hungrier and digest food more completely. Here are two herbs that can help increase your appetite:

Gentian. Herbalists usually recommend this traditional bitter (*Gentiana lutea*). Boil 1 teaspoon of dried, powdered root (available from health food stores and suppliers) in about 3 cups of water. You can drink two cups a day.

Quassia. This bitter herb, made from the bark of a tropical tree (*Picrasma excelsa*), is often used to treat anorexia. Boil 1 teaspoon of the crushed bark in 2 cups of water for ½ hour, and drink a cup a day.

HERBAL
Resources

HERB ORGANIZATIONS

American Botanical Council
P.O. Box 144345
Austin, TX 78714-4345
Phone: 512-926-4900; 800-373-7105
Fax: 512-926-2345
e-mail: abc@herbalgram.org
Web site: www.herbalgram.org
Publishes the quarterly HerbalGram
*magazine plus booklets and scientific
reprints.*

American Herb Association
P.O. Box 1673
Nevada City, CA 95959
Phone: 530-265-9552
Fax: 530-274-3140
Publishes the newsletter AHA Quarterly
*and source lists. This group, which focuses on
medicinal herbs, offers lists of resources, pub-
lic gardens, and herbal medicine schools.*

The Herb Society of America, Inc.
9019 Kirtland Chardon Road
Mentor, OH 44094
Phone: 216-256-0514
Fax: 216-256-0541
e-mail: herbsociet@aol.com
Web site: www.herbsociety.org
*Herb gardeners may want to check out
this society, which sponsors an herb garden
at the U.S. National Arboretum in
Washington, D.C.*

Herb Research Foundation
1007 Pearl Street, Suite 200
Boulder, CO 80302
Phone: 303-449-2265
Fax: 303-449-7849
e-mail: info@herbs.org
Web site: www.herbs.org
*The foundation encourages and dissem-
inates research on herbs, especially for
medicinal uses.*

MAIL-ORDER SUPPLIERS

Catalog prices change from year to
year. We suggest that you check the
phone, fax, or Web site before ordering
a catalog.

Bountiful Gardens
18001 Shafer Ranch Road
Willits, CA 95490
Phone: 707-459-6410
e-mail: bountiful@zapcom.net
Catalog free.

Companion Plants
7247 N. Coolville Ridge Road
Athens, OH 45701
Phone: 740-592-4643
Fax: 740-593-3092
e-mail: complants@frognet.net
Web site: www.frognet.net/
   companion_plants
*Catalog $3. More than 400 herb plants
and 120 seed types.*

Herbs-Liscious
1702 S. Sixth Street
Marshalltown, IA 50158
Phone: 515-752-4976
Fax: 515-753-5193
e-mail: herbs@marshallnet.com
Catalog $2. Herb plants, dried herbs, essential oils, special requests.

Horizon Herbs
P.O. Box 69
Williams, OR 97544
Phone: 541-846-6704
Fax: 541-846-6233
e-mail: herbseed@chatlink.com
Web site: www. chatlink.com/
   ~herbseed
Catalog free. Specializing in over 300 varieties of medicinal herb seeds and roots. Organically grown.

It's About Thyme
11726 Manchaca Road
Austin, TX 78748
Phone: 512-280-1192
Fax: 512-280-6356
e-mail: itsaboutthyme@msn.com
Catalog $1. Herbs include Southwestern varieties.

Nichols Garden Nursery
1190 North Pacific Highway
Albany, OR 97321-4580
Phone: 541-928-9280
Fax: 541-967-8406
e-mail: info@gardennursery.com
Web site: www.gardennursery.com
Catalog free. Herb seeds and supplies.

Richter's Herbs
357 Highway 47
Goodwood, Ontario, Canada L0C 1A0
Phone: 905-640-6677
Fax: 905-640-6641
e-mail: inquiry@richters.com
Web site: www.richters.com
Catalog free. Herb seeds and plants, dried herbs, essential oils, and books.

Sandy Mush Herb Nursery
316 Surrett Cove Road
Leicester, NC 28748-5517
Phone: 828-683-2014
Catalog $4. Wide selection of herb plants and seeds.

The Thyme Garden
20546 Alsea Highway
Alsea, OR 97324
Phone: 541-487-8671
Fax: 541-487-8671 (call first)
e-mail: thymegarden@proaxis.com
Web site: www.proaxis.com/~
   thymegarden
Catalog $2. Herb seeds, some plants and dried herbs.

Well-Sweep Herb Farm
205 Mt. Bethel Road
Port Murray, NJ 07865
Phone: 908-852-5390
Fax: 908-852-1649
Catalog $2. Herb plants, some seeds.

HERB PERIODICALS

The Business of Herbs, 439 Ponderosa Way, Jemez Springs, NM 87025.
Phone: 505-829-3448. Fax: 505-829-3449. e-mail: HerbBiz@aol.com

The Herb Companion, Interweave Press, 201 East Fourth Street, Dept. 0-B, Loveland, CO 80537-5655. Phone: 800-456-6018. Fax: 970-667-8317.
Web site: www.interweave.com/iwpsite/herbie/herbie/html
e-mail: custserv@herbalgram.org

HerbalGram, P.O. Box 144345, Austin, TX 78714-4345. Phone: 512-926-4900. e-mail: custserv@herbalgram.org

Herb Quarterly, P.O. Box 689, San Anselmo, CA 94960. Phone: 415-455-9540. Fax: 415-455-9541. e-mail: HerbQuart@aol.com

BOOKS ON HERBS

Bown, Deni. *Encyclopedia of Herbs & Their Uses.* New York: Dorling Kindersley, 1995. A heavily illustrated encyclopedia of herbs, including garden design, natural distribution of herbs and uses in their regions of origin, and medicinal applications.

Castleman, Michael. *The Healing Herbs.* Emmaus, PA: Rodale Press, 1991. Contains fascinating anecdotes about historical uses and lore, plus recent research, possible future uses, and advice on dosages.

Chevallier, Andrew. *The Encyclopedia of Medicinal Plants.* New York: Dorling Kindersley, 1996. This encyclopedia features a detailed history of herbal use and illustrates key preparations of medicinal herbs.

DeBaggio, Thomas. *Growing Herbs from Seed, Cutting & Root.* Loveland, CO: Interweave Press, 1994. By the owner of a popular herb nursery in Arlington, Virginia, this book will be helpful to anyone who is starting or expanding an herb garden.

Dodt, Colleen K. *The Essential Oils Book: Creating Personal Blends for Mind and Body.* Pownal, VT: Storey Books, 1996. A compendium of uses for essential oils including recipes and tips for herbal healing.

Duke, James A., Ph.D. *The Green Pharmacy.* Emmaus, PA: Rodale Press, 1997. With his signature blend of scientific knowledge and folk wisdom, Duke suggests simple concoctions and tactics for preventing and alleviating conditions that range from aging and altitude sickness to warts and worms.

Foster, Steven. *Echinacea: Nature's Immune Enhancer.* Rochester, VT: Healing Arts Press, 1991. A detailed, highly scientific examination of research and cultivation.

Foster, Steven. *Herbal Renaissance: Growing, Using & Understanding Herbs in the Modern World.* Salt Lake City, UT: Gibbs Smith Publisher, 1993. A detailed examination of more than 90 herbs, with helpful directions for cultivation, propagation, and harvesting.

Foster, Steven, and James A. Duke. *A Field Guide to Medicinal Plants: Eastern and Central North America.* Boston, MA: Houghton Mifflin, 1990. A guide to identifying nearly 500 traditional herbal plants in the wild.

Grieve, Mrs. M. *A Modern Herbal.* New York, NY: Dover Publications, 1971. 2 vols. Today's herbalists consider this a classic — and thorough — description of traditional herbal medicine uses.

Michalak, Patricia S. *Herbs.* Rodale's Successful Organic Gardening Series. Emmaus, PA: Rodale Press, 1993. Whether you grow herbs for food or medicine, you want to avoid using garden chemicals. Here's how to grow healthy herbs nature's way.

Smith, Miranda. *Your Backyard Herb Garden.* Emmaus, PA: Rodale Press, 1997. A guide to growing more than 50 herbs, with tips for companion planting, pests, and diseases.

Tyler, Varro E., Ph.D. *Herbs of Choice: The Therapeutic Use of Phytomedicinals.* Binghamton, NY: Haworth Press, 1994. A critical look at the scientific basis for medicinal uses of herbs.

Tyler, Varro E., Ph.D., *The Honest Herbal: A Sensible Guide to the Use of Herbs and Related Remedies,* 3rd ed. Binghamton, NY: Haworth Press, 1993. Like *Herbs of Choice,* this book is a scientist's conservative assessment of medicinal herbs and their applications.

Weiner, Michael A., and Janet A. Weiner. *Herbs That Heal.* Mill Valley, CA: Quantam Books, 1994. The California-based Weiners describe traditional uses and recent research on more than 220 medicinal herbs, with suggestions for preparation.

ACKNOWLEDGEMENTS

I could never have written this book without the help and inspiration of the indefatigable Jim Duke, who seems to have all the answers in his database or in his head. Thanks also to Gwen Steege, the world's most patient editor; eagle-eye technical advisor Mindy Green; Steven Foster, Jim Emerson, JoAnne Wilkins, David Ellis, Alice Bagwill, and Steven Dentali. Thanks to the Outer Banks bunch — Judy, Mike, and Kerry — for putting up with reference books on the beach towels; my son, Hart, for the Post-Its; and my husband, David, for all the things I've been too busy to mention.

Index

Page references in *italics* indicate illustrations;
page references in **bold** indicate tables.